MEDICAL PRACTICE MANAGEMENT

Body of Knowledge Review

Second Edition

VOLUME 1

Business Operations

Medical Group Management Association
102 Inverness Terrace East
Englewood, CO 80112-5306
877.275.6462
mgma.com

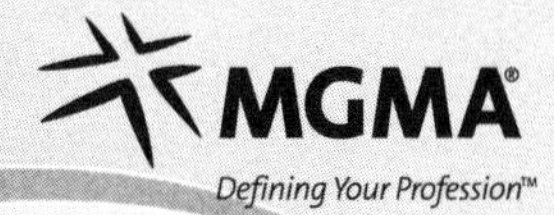

Medical Group Management Association® (MGMA®) publications are intended to provide current and accurate information and are designed to assist readers in becoming more familiar with the subject matter covered. Such publications are distributed with the understanding that MGMA does not render any legal, accounting, or other professional advice that may be construed as specifically applicable to an individual situation. No representations or warranties are made concerning the application of legal or other principles discussed by the authors to any specific factual situation, nor is any prediction made concerning how any particular judge, government official, or other person will interpret or apply such principles. Specific factual situations should be discussed with professional advisors.

PRODUCTION CREDITS
Publisher: Marilee E. Aust
Composition: Glacier Publishing Services, Inc.
Cover Design: Ian Serff, Serff Creative Group, Inc.

LIBRARY OF CONGRESS CATALOGING-IN-PUBLICATION DATA

Business operations.
p. ; cm. — (Medical practice management body of knowledge review (2nd ed.) ; v. 1)
Includes bibliographical references and index.
ISBN 978-1-56829-330-1
1. Medical offices—Management. I. Medical Group Management Association. II. Series.
[DNLM: 1. Practice Management, Medical—economics. W 80 B9789 2008]
R728.B886 2008
610.68—dc22

2008044466

Printed in the United States of America
10 9 8 7 6 5 4 3 2

Dedication

To our colleagues in the profession
of medical practice management
and to the groups that support us
in our efforts to serve our profession.

Body of Knowledge Review Series — Second Edition

VOLUME 1	Business Operations
VOLUME 2	Financial Management
VOLUME 3	Organizational Governance
VOLUME 4	Human Resource Management
VOLUME 5	Information Management
VOLUME 6	Patient Care Systems
VOLUME 7	Quality Management
VOLUME 8	Risk Management

Contents

Preface

TO SUCCEED AND FLOURISH in the day-to-day work environment of managing a medical practice, it is important that the successful administrator master and become adept at utilizing basic and advanced business operations skills.

The Business Operations domain within the *Medical Practice Management Body of Knowledge (BOK), second edition,* presents the basic building blocks needed to efficiently and effectively manage the day-to-day operations of a medical group practice, regardless of its legal or political structure. Included within the general competency of critical thinking skills, the Business Operations domain requires an in-depth understanding of the other competencies for the effective management of a group practice.

When faced with the task of assuming the leadership of a medical practice, the effective medical practice executive should properly utilize the basic tools of business operations to properly evaluate the issues affecting the organization. Through the proper application of these tools, the administrator will be able to prepare and implement the steps needed to place the organization on a firm footing for survival and growth. Examples of the organizational effects that result when these tools are put to proper use can be seen in many organizations and real life experiences.

Knowledge of the tools within the Business Operations domain and the way they interact with the other domains within the BOK affords the health care administrator the ability to provide the direction and leadership needed by his or her organization. These same tools are utilized in the day-to-day operation of a practice and assist the administrator in ensuring the continued growth and development of the organization.

Body of Knowledge Review Series Contributors

Geraldine Amori, PhD, ARM, CPHRM
Douglas G. Anderson, FACMPE
James A. Barnes, MBA
Fred Beck, JD
Jerry D. Callahan Jr., CPA
Anthony J. DiPiazza, CPA
David N. Gans, MSHA, FACMPE
Robert L. Garrie, MPA, RHIA
Edward Gulko, MBA, FACMPE, FACHE, LNHA
Kenneth T. Hertz, CMPE
Steven M. Hudson, CFP, CFS, CRPC
Jerry Lagle, MBA, CPA, FACMPE
Michael Landers
Gary Lewins, FACMPE, CPA, FHFMA
Ken Mace, MA, CMPE
Jeffrey Milburn, MBA, CMPE
Michael A. O'Connell, MHA, FACMPE, CHE
Dawn M. Oetjen, PhD, MHA
Reid M. Oetjen, PhD, MSHSA
Pamela E. Paustian, MSM, RHIA
David Peterson, MBA, FACMPE
Lisa H. Schneck, MSJ
Frederic R. Simmons Jr., CPA
Thomas E. Sisson, CPA
Donna J. Slovensky, PhD, RHIA, FAHIMA
Jerry M. Trimm, PhD, FHIMSS
Stephen L. Wagner, PhD, FACMPE
Lee Ann H. Webster, MA, CPA, FACMPE
Susan Wendling-Aloi, MPA, FACMPE
Warren C. White Jr., FACMPE
Lawrence Wolper, MBA, FACMPE, CMC
Lorraine C. Woods, FACMPE
James R. Wurts, FACMPE

Learning Objectives

AFTER READING THIS VOLUME, the medical practice executive will be able to accomplish the following tasks:

- Develop, implement, and monitor business operation plans;
- Develop, implement, and oversee systems for the purchase of materials and equipment;
- Manage facilities planning and maintenance activities to meet the organization's current and future needs;
- Manage the discernment process for identification and utilization of outsourced expertise and business partners; and
- Develop and implement a marketing and communication plan.

Vignette

The Exam Glove Question[1]

WHEN I LOOKED AT THE SHELVES in the supply closet, they were packed full of exam gloves. There were pink gloves and blue gloves, plain gloves and fancy gloves. We had every size one could imagine, sterile and nonsterile, latex and latex-free. When I asked why we had so many different gloves, I was told that a physician or staff member requested them. "Are we still using all of them?" I inquired.

"Oh, no. Many of the physicians and staff who requested certain gloves have either transferred to other locations or no longer work for the clinic."

I asked what happens to the gloves that no one uses.

"We just push them to the back of the shelf until someone asks for them."

"Oh," I said. I could only wonder what the supply closets looked like in our five other locations.

Are You Wasting Money on Inventory? In Other Areas?

My encounter with the exam gloves prompted me to think about just how many of our resources were tied up in unnecessary supply inventory and how wasteful it was to have such a large selection of exam gloves. Not only did we have a large inventory, but we also incurred the cost of ordering the gloves – and we paid more for them because we ordered such small quantities. If we managed our gloves like that, it was likely that we managed many other areas in a similar manner.

One of the principles of quality improvement is standardization. That means doing things the same way, having the same policies, and using the same supplies from location to location and department to department. It involves removing variation. That includes work processes, supplies, policies, forms, and, yes, exam gloves.

The clinic I work for has designated leaders at each location. We had developed consistent personnel policies and a staff performance and compensation plan. However, we had no consistency in operating policies, forms, supplies, and patient flow. We faced the challenge of removing the inefficiencies and inconsistencies from the system. The question was how.

Standardize to Save Time, Money, and Effort

We started the standardization process by agreeing on its benefits. We needed that foundation and vision to help us through the process. Commitment and buy-in was critical. However, change just didn't happen on its own. We had to bring together the leaders from each clinic location and build a team to oversee the process. Although the individuals were acquainted with one another, they did not perceive themselves as a team. Most of the time, they functioned independently. Locations shared information, but we had no mechanism to develop a consistent method that would apply to all of them.

To remedy that, clinic leaders started meeting on a regular basis to discuss how to approach the project. We used Patrick Lencioni's book, *The Five Dysfunctions of a Team*,[2] to help us learn to overcome our impaired behaviors and work together more closely. We practiced those skills. We identified specific areas of focus, including supplies, operating policies, forms, and patient flow. We established work groups for each area, which analyzed existing processes and made suggestions for improvement.

One of the most powerful recommendations came from the Forms Committee. We had hundreds of forms – often multiple forms for the same purpose. The Forms Committee was able to standardize forms from location to location and eliminate a significant number of duplications. It also made forms available on the clinic's intranet so staff could complete them online and print them. The result: a significant savings on printing and inventory costs.

Valuable (Thrifty) Lessons

What did we learn? First, standardization takes time and persistent effort. It's an ongoing process. Second, the necessary team building strengthens the organization and prepares it for future group challenges. Third, standardization is great preparation for implementing an electronic health record (EHR).

We began our EHR implementation in March. Our standardization approach extends to training; equipment, such as tablet computers; guidelines for problem lists; the transfer of data from paper charts; and entering data into the system as patients are cared for. At the same time we are allowing some flexibility for physicians and providers to use the system in a way that fits their work style.

My challenge to you: Take a look at your supply closet and see just how many types of exam gloves are on the shelf.

Current Business Operations Issues

WHEN LOOKING at the Business Operations domain from a broad perspective, it is clear that this domain is in a state of change. It is apparent that the domain is in a state of evolution as it attempts to maintain balance while also changing to meet the demands and expectations of the individual stakeholders as well as society as a whole. The practice administrator should take the time to identify and understand the specific pressures of operations as well as those issues that are core within other domains but also affect this domain.

Numerous internal and external pressures affect the operational side of practice management. These pressures include, but are not limited to:

1. Regulatory changes at the federal, state, and local levels;
2. Third-party payer demands and expectations;
3. Patient demands and expectations;
4. Staff, physician, and community expectations; and last but not least,
5. Aligning the business plan with the practice's mission and strategic plan.

Other key issues that affect the operational areas are well represented in other domains. These issues include:

1. The effect of the Health Insurance Portability and Accountability Act of 1996 regulation;
2. The ability to recruit and retain qualified staff; and
3. The need to control costs in a variety of areas, including staffing, supplies, regulatory demands, third-party contracting, and information management.

Knowledge Needs

TO PROPERLY AND EFFECTIVELY RESPOND to the ongoing internal and external forces on both the practice and business of medicine, the medical practice executive should be well grounded in the fundamentals of day-to-day operations and the methodologies needed to maintain and improve the processes that affect organizations during these ever-evolving times. Expertise in these fundamental business and clinical skills is the ultimate goal. Several of the key skills include the ability to use project management techniques to measure and improve practice operations; the development and implementation of survey techniques to identify expectations and perceived shortcomings among various user groups; and the identification of organizational needs while evaluating, designing, and implementing changes to meet those needs. Finally, the practice executive needs to know how the various parts of the operation fit together and how they complement and support each other.

Business operations includes five distinct tasks, as identified in each chapter in this volume. Each task is interconnected with the others through several strong, identifiable threads, namely:

1. Analyzing how an organization accomplishes its tasks with an eye toward change;
2. Bringing all stakeholders into the process to ensure that everyone's needs are met in an effective and efficient manner without endangering others' needs;

3. Maintaining attention to detail – many tasks allow viewing the situation as a "big picture," but these tasks also require the administrator to ensure that all of the dots and dashes are in the right places;
4. Communicating the changes and improvements that are implemented to provide quality care and meet patient needs in a cost-effective manner.

Chapter 1 Operational Planning

TO BE EFFECTIVE in today's market, medical group practices should adopt some of the same tools used in other successful "businesses," including strategic plans, marketing plans, and business plans. Whereas the strategic plan tends to focus on trends and competition, a business plan addresses the practice's resources, such as the breadth and depth of the practice, technological expertise, and service delivery capabilities, among other assets. The marketing plan, which is separate from business plans, focuses on customers – patients, other physicians and groups, payers, vendors, and the community at large.

Selecting a Plan

There are four basic types of business plans, each with a unique purpose and audience:

1. Start-up business plan;
2. Ongoing financial business plan;
3. Operational business plan; and
4. Bank-financing plan.

Start-up Business Plan

Practices that are seeking funds to help start a new venture, such as opening a second office or purchasing equipment to offer new services, need to complete a start-up business plan (also known as a feasibility plan). This type of plan is used to convince potential investors to provide the practice with the necessary capital to pursue this new venture. A start-up plan is sometimes referred to as an "idea" plan. In this type of plan, the practice would brainstorm and then outline the venture: What problem, weakness, or opportunity is the practice addressing through this plan? How does this new venture solve the problem? Why is this solution better than others? How will it be marketed? What resources are required to make it happen? The purpose of this type of plan is to allow the practice to see whether the venture is worth undertaking. If so, the practice can use the plan to recruit stakeholders who share its vision and bring them on board for the new venture.

Ongoing Financial Business Plan

Established practices that are seeking financial support may complete an ongoing financial business plan. This type of plan will also allow potential lending sources to view the practice's ongoing financial status, risk, past and future spending habits, and prospects before committing funds. Because the practice is established, financials from more than one year can be trended.

Operational Business Plan

A third type of plan is the operational business plan, the most detailed of the plans. It documents exact operation plans for the practice through items such as the detailed operating budget, detailed market and competitor research and analysis, product design specification, sales prospect lists, partner acquisition strategies, intellectual property strategies, and anything else that guides the group's growth.

Bank-Financing Plan

The final type of business plan is the bank-financing plan, used when a practice is trying to obtain a bank loan. Perhaps the group would like to offer a new ancillary service that requires significant capital (e.g., lab services, radiology, etc.). Bank funding is usually available only if the practice either has a solid operating history with positive cash flows or can put up collateral to cover the loan (for a start-up, this means something of great value, such as a house).

The bank-financing plan focuses on persuading the banker that the practice can satisfy these needs through historical financial ratios, assets, and so forth.

Getting Started

Before writing a business plan, the medical practice executive should consider four core questions:

1. **What** service or product does the practice provide and what needs does it fill?
2. **Who** are the potential customers for the practice's service(s) and why will they choose the practice for them?
3. **How** will the practice reach its potential customers?
4. **Where** will the practice get the financial resources to start new endeavors, such as new products or services?

The preparation of a written business plan is not the end result of the planning process. The realization of that plan is the ultimate goal. However, the writing of the plan is an important intermediate stage – *fail to plan can mean plan to fail*. For an established practice, it demonstrates that careful consideration has been given to the practice's development; and for a start-up, it shows that the entrepreneur has done his or her homework.

A formal business plan is just as important for an established practice, irrespective of its size, as it is for a start-up practice. It serves four critical functions:

1. Helps a practice to clarify, focus, and research its planned future development and prospects.
2. Provides a considered and logical framework within which a practice can develop and pursue business strategies over the next three to five years.
3. Serves as a basis for discussion with third parties such as shareholders, agencies, banks, and investors.
4. Offers a benchmark against which actual practice performance can be measured and reviewed.

Business Plan Components

Five main components are typically found in every business plan: (1) an executive summary, (2) a business section, (3) a market analysis section, (4) a financial section, and (5) a management section.

Executive Summary

Every business plan begins with an executive summary. The executive summary is the "first impression" of the practice that you give to the reader, be it a potential lender, partner, or investor. The cliché "You never have a second chance to make a good first impression" applies here because the success of the plan can often depend on the executive summary. The executive summary briefly, yet accurately, responds to the five core questions – the who, what, when, where, and how of the venture. It also provides a succinct overview of each of the other main components of the plan (e.g., business, market analysis, financials, and management) as well as components from the strategic plan (mission, vision, values, goals, and objectives). The executive summary answers the questions: Where is the practice going? What will it look like when it gets there? What is the present situation in the community (and for larger groups – across the country) and how does it affect the practice? What is the status of the practice's products or services? What about its finances? What management is in place? Who needs to be hired or recruited? The executive summary should be written *after* the business plan has been completed.

Business Section

The second component of the business plan is the business section. This section discusses the practice's structure, management, staffing, operations, and business relationships. This section usually begins with a brief description of the industry as it looks today, as well as how it will look in the future. Information on all the various markets within the industry, including any new products or developments that will benefit or adversely affect the practice, should also be discussed. An explanation of the structure – general or limited partnership, sole proprietorship, or corporation, for example – should be stated, as well as the practice's legal form, who its principals are, and what they will bring to the venture.

After the description of the practice's business comes an explanation of the products or services the practice intends to market. The products/services description statement should be complete enough to give a clear idea of the practice's intentions. Emphasis should be given to any unique features or variations from concepts that can typically be found in the industry. Examples of where a practice's unique features can be promoted might include sponsoring a booth at a county fair providing free blood pressure and cholesterol screening, or physicians attending disease-specific support groups (congenital heart, diabetes, etc.) and providing information and, often more importantly, answering patient and family member's questions.

Market Analysis Section

The next section of the business plan provides a market analysis, which is essentially a summary of the practice's marketing plan. The market analysis demonstrates the demand for the practice's products or services, the proposed market, and trends within the industry. In addition, it describes the practice's pricing plan and policies. This section helps the practice understand and define its market, the demographics and psychographics of its target customers, competitor's products or services, and both business and environmental risks.

For marketing to be effective, the medical group practice should have a differentiable market position that can be held out to the potential client in a verifiable, demonstrable way. Marketing activities in a business plan must be based on a foundation of practice management activities to truly differentiate the practice.[3] Practice management activities in a business plan include steps such as increasing the practice's patient base or capabilities through recruiting additional physicians, developing new products or services, developing in-depth industry knowledge (by which the practice will be known as being expert within a particular specialty), and so forth.[4]

The world might "beat a path to your door," but only if people know who you are, what you've got, and where to find you. Thus, the market analysis also includes the practice's advertising and promotion, pricing and profitability, selling tactics, distribution, public relations, and business relationships.[5] A key component of the market analysis section that affects everything the practice does throughout its business is summarized in the question: How will the practice use an investor's money to efficiently market to its customers?

Financial Section

The next section of the business plan comprises the financials of the practice. This section demonstrates that the practice is as committed to its business venture as it expects those reading the business plan to be. The practice's capital requirements and profit potential are analyzed and demonstrated here. This is accomplished through numerous financial statements, often based on a modified accrual accounting system that also takes into consideration "noncash" items (e.g., capital expenditures, such as equipment or building leases). This is done in an effort to best reflect the financial health of the practice.

Accounting Methods

Accrual-based accounting systems record financial situations based on events that change the net worth of the practice (the amount owed to the practice less the amount the practice owes others). Standard practice is to record and recognize revenues when they become available and measurable (i.e., known). The term "available" means collectible within the current period or soon enough thereafter to be used to pay the liabilities of the current period. Expenditures, if measurable, are recorded in the accounting period in which the liabilities are incurred. An exception is unmatured interest on general long-term debt, which should be recorded when it is due.

This differs from cash-based accounting, used less often in medical practice management. In cash-based accounting, income and expenses are recognized only when cash is received or paid out. Cash-based accounting also defers all credit transactions to a later date. It is more conservative for the practice in that it does not record revenue until cash receipt. In a growing practice this results in a lower income bottom line compared to accrual-based accounting.

Financial statements should be prepared on the modified accrual basis to show the amount and source of personal funds the practice is contributing, the amount of capital needed, and the practice's plan to repay this debt. All pertinent financial worksheets should be included in this section: income statement, a break-even worksheet, projected cash flow statements, and a balance sheet. A review of the practice's return on investment and discounted cash-flow value should also be completed.

Income Statement

The income statement is a report on the proposed or current business's cash-generating ability. The income statement illustrates just how much the practice makes or loses during the year by subtracting cost of goods and expenses from revenue to arrive at a net result – which is either a profit or a loss. For a business plan, the income statement should be generated on a monthly basis during the first year, quarterly for the second, and annually for each year thereafter. Following the income statement is a note analyzing the statement. The analysis statement should be very short, emphasizing key points within the income statement.[6]

Break-Even Worksheet

The break-even worksheet computes the break-even point and sales level needed to earn a given profit by analyzing relationships between fixed costs, variable costs per unit, quantity, price, and profit. This calculation is completed by first filling in all of the practice's expected fixed monthly expenses; these are expenses that will not change, regardless of the amount of services provided (how much is "sold"). These will add up to the practice's total fixed costs. The next step is to divide the total monthly fixed costs by the gross profit per unit. The result of this calculation is the break-even point.

The practice will operate at a loss until it reaches the break-even point (that is, total costs = total revenues).

Cash Flow Statement

The cash flow statement shows how much cash will be needed to meet obligations, when it is going to be required, and what the source will be. It shows a schedule of the money coming into the practice and expenses that need to be paid out. The result is the profit or loss at the end of the month or year. If the practice runs a loss on its cash flow statement, it is a strong indicator that the practice will need additional cash to meet expenses.[7]

The cash flow statement also should be prepared on a monthly basis during the first year, on a quarterly basis during the second year, and on an annual basis thereafter. As with the income statement, the cash flow statement should be presented in a short summary in the business plan covering the key points derived from the cash flow statement.[8]

Balance Sheet

The last financial statement needed for the business plan is the balance sheet. Like the income and cash flow statements, the balance sheet uses information from all of the financial models developed in earlier sections of the business plan; however, unlike the previous statements, the balance sheet is generated solely on an annual basis for the business plan and is, more or less, a summary of all the preceding financial information broken down into three areas: (1) assets; (2) liabilities; and (3) equity.[9]

Assets are classified as current, long-term, or fixed. Current assets are those that will be converted to cash or will be used by the practice in a year or less, including cash, accounts receivable, inventory, and supplies. Long-term assets are those that will last more than one year, such as capital equipment, property, and investments. Fixed assets are similar to long-term assets, and include property, building structures, and so forth.

Like assets, liabilities are classified as current or long term. If the debts are due in one year or less, they are classified as current liabilities; if they are due in more than one year, they are long-term liabilities. Examples of current liabilities are accounts payable, accrued liabilities, and taxes; long-term liabilities include payables in the forms of bonds, notes, and mortgages.

The final portion of the balance sheet is the practice's equity, which is the difference between its total assets and total liabilities. The amount of equity the practice has is used by investors when evaluating the company to determine the amount of capital they think they can safely invest in the business.

In the business plan, an analysis statement for the balance sheet should be created just as was done for the income and cash flow statements. The analysis of the balance sheet should be kept short and cover key points about the practice.

Return on Investment and Discounted Cash Flow

Two types of valuation methods typically found in business plans include return on investment (ROI) and discounted cash flow. ROI is a measure of the practice's ability to use its assets to generate additional value for shareholders. It is used to determine whether a proposed investment is reasonable and how well this investment will repay the shareholder. It is calculated as the ratio of the amount gained (net profit or net loss) divided by net worth and expressed as a percentage. If a group practice has immediate objectives such as getting market revenue share, building infrastructure, or positioning itself for sale, an ROI might be measured in terms of meeting one or more of these objectives rather than in immediate profit or cost saving.

Discounted cash flow expresses how much a practice is worth today based on what it will earn in the future. It informs shareholders of their expected rate of return, given the amount invested and the practice's financial projections, and how much equity they will receive for the investment. It is a fairly accurate measure because it discounts, or adjusts, cash flows (projected ups and downs of revenue over a period of time) by a rate that is acceptable to the shareholder to account for risk and the time the investor must wait for a return.

Each of these methods is valuable to the business plan. The underlying idea of these valuation methods is that money today is worth more than money a year, or five years, or ten years, and so on, from now because money in hand can be invested to earn interest and there is no risk you may not receive it in the future; it follows the adage "time value of money."

Risk Tolerance

The risk tolerance of the practice – its attitude toward accepting risk – plays a significant role in its financial planning. Risk tolerance is not something that can be measured, but asking a few questions can help the practice determine whether it is conservative, moderate, or aggressive in its financial makeup. A practice that is unfamiliar with investing, fearful of asset loss, or prefers saving to investing could be classified as having a rather conservative tolerance for risk. Conversely, a practice that is comfortable with long-term goal investing, that can withstand short-term losses, and that is also comfortable with the turbulent nature of investing is aggressively risk tolerant. A practice that is somewhat in the middle of these extremes is classified as moderately risk tolerant.

Shareholders also vary in their levels of risk tolerance and want to be compensated for their risk; sound financial management and planning, along with the use of valuation strategies, allow this to occur.

Management Section

A discussion of the practice's management is the final piece of its business plan. This includes a description of the practice's organizational structure and administrative team (including resumes and biographies) as well as staffing projection data for the near future.

The goal of this section is to demonstrate how the practice and its administration are uniquely qualified and capable of achieving success. In particular, the following questions should be answered: Can the practice relate to the community and draw customers for its services from it? Can the practice deliver what these customers really want? Is the practice's administrative team qualified to do this?

The management section of the business plan is really a mini-interview with the practice's administration to assure an investor, lender, or potential partner that it has lined up the right people to make the venture a success. This section is one of the most crucial of the entire business plan. The only thing that will ensure success is the day-to-day activity of qualified people who are in the "driver's seat" following a mapped plan toward a vision.[10]

Summary

A business plan should be a realistic view of the expectations and long-term objectives for an established practice or a new venture to be undertaken by the practice. It provides the framework within which the practice must operate and, ultimately, succeed or fail. For a medical practice seeking external support, the plan is the most important sales document it is ever likely to produce because it could be the key to raising finances. Preparation of a comprehensive plan will not guarantee success in raising funds or mobilizing support, but lack of a sound plan will, almost certainly, ensure failure.[11]

Facilitating Business Planning

"Planning is a process by which management visualizes the future and develops specific courses of action to achieve organizational goals."[12] To set a proper foundation for the business operations planning process, it is important to first set a strategic framework plan and clearly articulate the organization's mission, vision, and values.

Strategic planning seeks to formulate those organizational goals and plans that normally take five to ten years to accomplish. Strategic planning also requires the administrator to take a long-term view of the organizational environment and base plans on the present business environment, and it demands that the planning be constantly updated to evolve and respond to the ever-changing external and internal dynamics. The *strategic plan* is therefore a dynamic document that must be constantly updated.

The *mission statement* defines the unique and distinctive purpose of the organization. It should be succinct and to the point without promising something that the organization cannot provide or prove, such as a statement that the organization provides the "highest" level of care in the area. In summary, the mission statement should state who the organization is and what it is about.

To determine where the organization needs to grow or change in the future, it is helpful to create a *vision statement*. Whereas the mission statement conveys what the organization is today, the vision statement communicates what the organization wants to be in the future. Although this statement is normally the "dream" of the organization, it should have a basis in reality or it will become irrelevant to both the staff within the organization and anyone else desirous of learning about the goals of the organization.

The last document used to create the planning framework is the *values statement.* The values statement defines the culture of the organization and, by doing so, clearly states the ethics and principles that guide the organization and all of its members.[13]

Operational, or tactical, planning addresses the more immediate, short-term needs of an organization and supports or complements the strategic plan. Operational planning includes such issues as planning for staff vacation coverage or developing a budget for the next year. Because operational plans have a much shorter life span, they are not as affected as strategic plans by changes in external and internal dynamics. The importance of operational planning is to create a foundation that can be used by departments and other components of the organization to develop their own plans and budgets. The development of these operational plans should take into account the mission and vision of the organization as well as the resources that are available to meet the plans and goals of the organization. This operational or tactical plan, in addressing short-term or relatively immediate issues, should include several components, such as:

1. Identifying and defining the problem or issue to be addressed;
2. Identifying the goal that will define the completion of this plan as a success;
3. Identifying the resources (e.g., personnel, equipment, supplies, space, and funding) needed to complete the plan;
4. Determining the time line for competing the plan; and
5. Identifying the potential interactions with other stakeholders and affected parties.

For planning to work, the strategies and tactics to be employed must be consistent with the culture of the organization. The culture of the organization sets the tone for how the organization will project itself to the outside world as well as how it will act internally from an operational perspective and through interactions among the various staff and providers. This culture both emanates from and is affected by the goals, perspectives, background, and ethics of the leadership in addition to the impact of the demographics and expectations of the surrounding community in which the practice is located. Developing the culture necessary for supportive buy-in requires proactive initiatives by the physician as well as the administrative leadership. The development of the values statement that was previously discussed is helpful in identifying the internal culture of the organization. The organization's culture should also acknowledge and be responsive to any individual cultural barriers or differences that may exist among the various stakeholders of the organization.

Whenever change is being contemplated within an organization, there often is concern. Some of this concern emanates from the physicians, who are not always able to understand the difference between the practice of medicine and the business of health care. Physicians become proficient in the practice of medicine during residencies and fellowships, but practice managers should help physicians understand and come to grips with the requirements, and often conflicting demands, of the business of health care. For example, an orthopedic physician may want to add radiology services to the practice without first conducting feasibility plans or formally assessing the opportunity by looking at the community's ability to support the service. It is the manager's responsibility to explain and show physicians why the operations and strategic plans including (or not including) such opportunities are important and appropriate for the practice's future.

Through the use of management-led working committees, supervisory councils, and staff meetings, physicians and staff will become more understanding of, and comfortable with, the structure of the operations plan. Through such education, physicians and staff can become integral parts of the planning process, thereby helping to evolve and grow a corporate culture that embraces both planning and change.

Chapter 2 Developing and Purchasing Materials and Equipment

THE PURCHASING SYSTEM IS A KEY COMPONENT in the operation of any medical practice. It determines how well medical groups can get the right goods and services in the right place, at the right time, for the right price, and in the most efficient and effective way possible.

All operating costs or overhead except for W-2 employees' salaries and related payroll taxes are "purchasing system processed costs" and go through the practice's purchasing function. In addition, many groups make large expenditures for fixed assets; these costs reside on the practice's balance sheet until they are transferred to the income statement as operating costs through depreciation.

According to the Medical Group Management Association's (MGMA's) *Cost Survey, 2008 Report Based on 2007 Data,* the median operating costs for multispecialty practices, and most non-hospital-based single-specialty practices, range from $172,000 to $245,000 per full-time-equivalent physician.[14] These costs account for 31 percent to 38 percent of the group's total revenue.[15] For practices with extensive lab and outpatient treatment services, the costs can be much higher. The same *Cost Survey Report for 2008 based on 2007 Data* shows that the median purchasing system processed costs for hematology and oncology practices are approximately $2,800,000, or about 60 percent of total revenue.[16] Finally, these amounts and percentages are even higher when provider costs (except for compensation and payroll taxes) are included in purchasing system processed costs.

Major cost line items in purchasing system processed costs include:

- Drug supplies;
- Medical and surgical supplies;
- Building and occupancy costs;
- Furniture and equipment;
- Administrative supplies and services;
- Clinical labs;
- Radiology and imaging costs;
- Management fees; and
- Employee benefits.

Understanding a practice's purchasing function requires a working knowledge of the overall purchasing cycle, which is depicted in Exhibit 1.

Most medical practice business systems that account for a large amount of revenues or expenses are somewhat centralized in the practice, and physician-owners (or at least the administrators) play a critical role in their oversight and review. The segregation of oversight duties between owner and administrator is important to maintaining a strong internal control system. For example, billing system activities are usually initiated by physicians documenting their services and coding their own charges. Often, the physician-owners have a keen interest in reviewing the billing and collection reports because the content of these reports directly affects the physician's compensation.

The payroll system in most medical practices operates under a strict set of accounting controls; these include approval of pay rates and hours worked, security of internal or outsourced payroll processing, and payroll check review signatures by the administrator or physician-owner.

EXHIBIT 1
Purchasing Cycle

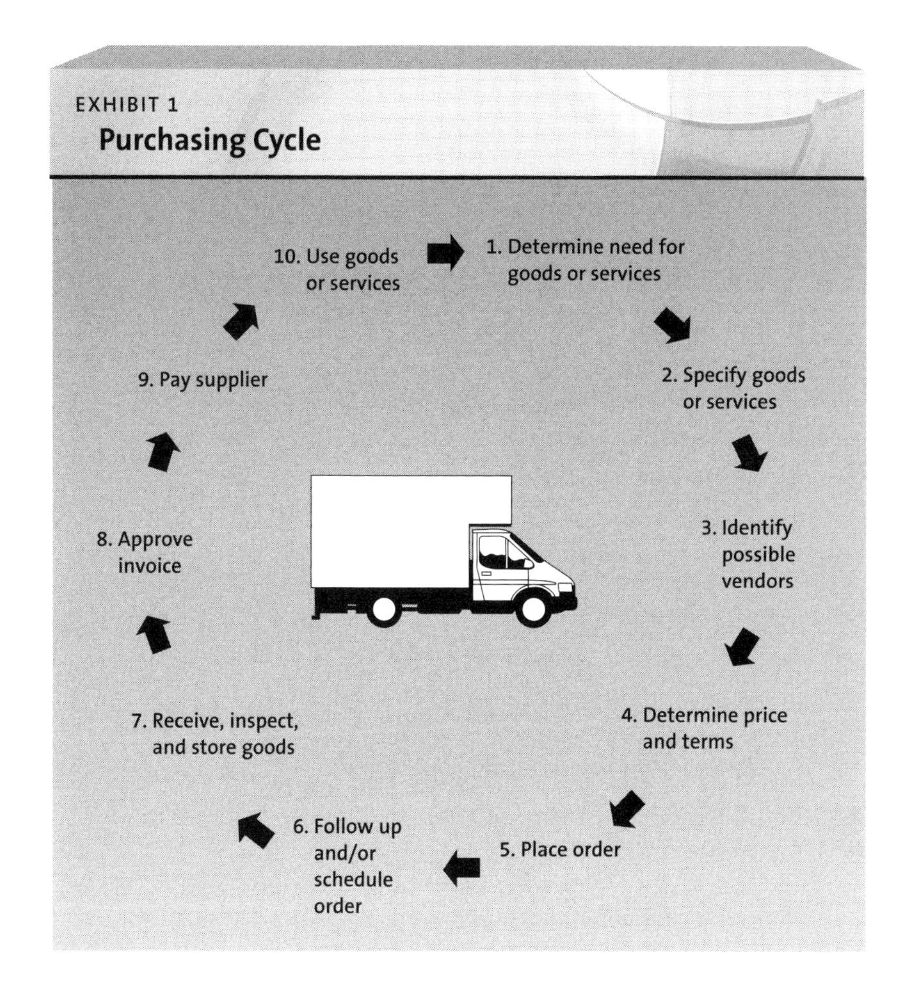

Other business systems are tightly controlled and have a high degree of executive oversight. In addition, these systems have detailed written policies and procedures.

In many medical practices, the purchasing function is decentralized and fragmented throughout an organization, with responsibility assigned to both clinical and administrative staff. Critical day-to-day details such as ordering and receiving goods and services are often delegated to low-level employees, with minimal oversight required. A recent study of spending behavior of physicians revealed that in medical practices with 4.0 to 5.9 practicing physicians, the ordering

EXHIBIT 2

Supply and Capital Expenditure Purchasing Decisions by Position

Position	Medical / Surgical Supplies	Capital Expenditure[17]
Practice Administrator / CEO	23.1%	53.9%
Nurses	33.3%	0.0%
Office / Clinic manager	20.5%	5.1%
Administrative assistant	6.4%	0.0%
Health system personnel	7.7%	1.3%
Board of directors or board committee	0.0%	25.6%
Purchasing director / Manager / Clerk	5.1%	0.0%
Physician	1.3%	12.8%
All others	2.6%	1.3%
	100.0%	100.0%

decisions for medical and surgical supplies and capital expenditures were made by employees in the positions shown in Exhibit 2.

Purchasing policies and procedures are rarely documented and reviewed. In fact, many practices do not even have written purchasing policies.

Most medical practices are small businesses with a limited staff. Typically they do not have purchasing departments and generally lack significant purchasing expertise. Very large practices and integrated delivery systems, however, do have sophisticated purchasing departments.

The following sections describe each step of the purchasing process and identify potential financial and operating risks. They conclude with recommendations for practices to consider in improving their purchasing functions.

1. **Determine the Need for Goods and Services**

   Determining the need for goods and services is often the responsibility of the end user. For example, nurses and medical assistants determine what exam room equipment and supplies they need.

For new services, the manager initiating the service usually identifies what supplies are needed. Equipment and other supply companies can help determine what is needed to implement a new service. The manager can also ask colleagues who provide a similar service what supplies and services they use.

For ongoing services, it is important to determine whether the practice's current supply list provides the best result to the patient at the most reasonable cost. Over time, new products and services enter the market that deliver comparable or better results at a lower cost. Sometimes natural resource costs, patent expirations, or private label alternatives provide a comparable or better alternative at a lower price than the practice's current supply item. Practices should periodically review their supply list for ongoing services.

Recommendation summary:

- Consult with supply companies and other practices in determining what goods and services you need; and
- Periodically review the supply and service list to determine if current supplies are providing the highest level of quality and the best value.

2. Specify Goods or Services

Once the needed goods or services have been identified, a practice must specify, in detail, the goods or services to be ordered. Some practices use a standard order form known as a purchase order or purchase requisition. Purchase orders normally contain the following information:

- Date of purchase order;
- Purchase order number;
- Originator's name, department, and contact information;
- A complete and very detailed description of the goods or services;
- Quantity;

- Price;
- Date needed;
- Shipping address;
- Billing address; and
- Any special shipping instructions.

It is important to remember purchasing controls such as requests for proposal, standing orders, and group purchasing.

While few practices actually use purchase orders because of the administrative burden, standard purchase orders can help ensure that goods and services are properly specified and delivered promptly. Precise specifications are critical for many clinical supplies.

Recommendation summary:

- Specify, in detail, what goods and services are to be ordered;
- Consider using standard prenumbered purchase orders; and
- Ask vendors about opportunities to make purchases online for ease and efficiency.

3. Identify Potential Vendors

Once a practice has determined what it needs and has described the goods and services and delivery requirements in detail, it must seek out possible vendors. Potential vendors can be identified through a variety of sources; these include:

- Current suppliers;
- Equipment manufacturers;
- Other practices;
- Hospitals;
- Trade associations;
- The Internet; and
- Telephone book yellow pages.

Practices should keep a list of and maintain contact with many backup vendors for the same goods and services in case the practice's primary dealer is unable to deliver. Group purchasing organizations (GPOs) are also a very good source of potential vendors; these organizations negotiate deals for the purchase of medical goods and services on behalf of their members, which include hospitals, nursing homes, medical practices, and other provider organizations.

Recommendation summary:

- Identify as many vendors as possible;
- Use all reasonable sources to identify potential vendors;
- Maintain relationships with several backup vendors; and
- Consider using GPOs.

4. Determine Price and Terms

Once a practice has determined its needs, specified the goods or services in detail, and identified all possible qualified vendors, it must negotiate the price to be paid and the terms.

Negotiating and maintaining the best price and terms may be the most critical step in the purchasing cycle. But it is often the task for which medical practices are the least prepared. Physicians and administrators have very little training and are uncomfortable in negotiating. As noted earlier, it is frequently an entry-level clinical employee who is tasked with ordering supplies and services and negotiating their price.

Medical equipment and other supply companies employ highly trained sales professionals whose compensation is directly proportional to the dollar volume of goods sold and the profitability of each account. With all the training and experience that these sales professionals have, it is no wonder that medical assistants, medical technicians, nurses, administrators, and even physicians are no match for these marketing warriors. Perhaps the most successful way to get the best value for the practice is to pit these sales gladiators against one another through periodically soliciting competitive bids for all goods and services.

Implementing a competitive bidding process is not difficult. The first step is to list the items the practice buys for the type of goods and services it provides. A Microsoft® *Excel* spreadsheet is a great tool for compiling and manipulating such a list. If the practice currently buys from a small number of vendors, it can usually get a report of purchases over the last year from each vendor that shows detailed product descriptions, manufacturers, and volume. Many vendors will provide the list in a spreadsheet format. If a practice uses more than one vendor, it will have to combine the vendor lists.

Even if the practice cannot secure a vendor list, it can build its own list by reviewing past invoices. If a complete list of purchases would take too long to develop, a list of the highest dollar volume items is usually sufficient. Often, practices find that a very limited number of items make up the majority of their purchases.

After the lists are developed, the practice calls a meeting (a bidders meeting) of all interested vendors identified in Step 3. This meeting is an effective way to communicate to the sales representative of each vendor that the practice is serious about implementing a competitive bidding process. At the meeting, the practice should distribute the supply bid list, provide any special shipping and billing requirements (by department or location), set a deadline for receiving the written bids (usually two weeks), and answer any questions the vendors may have. The practice may require the bidders to provide the bids in the same spreadsheet format as the practice is using. Answering vendor questions in a public forum like a bidders meeting will ensure that all vendors get the same information. If the practice must provide information to a particular vendor after the meeting, it should make sure that all bidders receive the same information.

When the bids come back from the vendors, their prices can be inserted in the spreadsheet. Prior-year quantities can be multiplied by the new prices to project the supply costs for the coming year for each of the vendors. If the spreadsheet includes the prior-year prices, the practice can compare the costs from the competitive bidding process to the actual cost paid the prior year.

This competitive bidding process can be repeated as often as the practice wishes. It is prudent to rebid the prices at least every year or two.

As noted earlier, the pricing component of the purchasing cycle is one of the most important for a practice. Not only are most practices ill prepared to match up with seasoned, aggressive sales people, it is probably one of the biggest risk areas for fraud and irregularities. The practice must be careful about delegating purchasing authority to those employees who lack negotiating skills. Sales people often woo these key decision makers with small gratuities such as movie passes, sporting event tickets, or gift cards to ensure their loyalty and convince them not to seek competitive bids or change vendors. In extreme cases, employees with purchasing authority may work in collusion with vendors, taking bribes or kickbacks, which could cost the practice thousands of dollars.

The control environment is an important consideration when evaluating a practice's purchasing cycle. A doctor or administrator accepting gifts, gratuities, and other favors from pharmaceutical company representatives, insurance agents, or major equipment vendors sets the wrong example for the practice's employees and sends the message that it is permissible to accept these favors.

The practice's leaders must set an ethical and moral example for their employees. In addition, purchasing policies and procedures should be established so that unprepared or unethical employees are not in a position to make major purchasing decisions without review. These policies should clearly prohibit physicians and employees from accepting gifts or gratuities from any supply company.

Recommendation summary:

- Establish purchasing policies and procedures with appropriate involvement and oversight by the practice's owners and leaders;
- Provide negotiating and purchasing training to those employees involved in the purchasing process;
- Create a positive control environment with segregation of duties, ethical training, and practice leaders that set an ethical example for employees;
- Adopt policies that prohibit employees from accepting gifts or gratuities from suppliers;
- Engage in a competitive bidding process whenever possible; and
- Solicit new bids for goods and services every year or two.

5. Place the Order

Another important step in the purchasing cycle is determining how much to order and when to place the order. A practice must make sure it has an adequate inventory of supplies on hand to fill the needs of its patients and providers.

Ordering, distribution, and supply chain managers have used the latest technology to significantly reduce the time between placing an order and delivery of that order. In addition, vendors offer expedited delivery systems if a practice finds itself running short on supplies.

Sometimes vendors provide great discounts for volume purchases. The challenge here is that medical practices seldom have a great deal of storage space. If discounts are significant, practices should consider acquiring additional space to store a greater volume of supplies.

Medical groups have to be very practical about their ordering steps. Many groups will order supplies, using an ordering calendar, at regular intervals such as weekly, biweekly, or monthly. An effective way to alert the practice when supply levels are low is simply to make a brightly colored mark in the practice's storage area: when the stock is depleted to the point that the bright mark is exposed, it is time to reorder.

Another important step in the ordering process relates back to the internal control environment. To prevent the relationship between the purchaser and the vendor from getting too personal, practices should rotate the person who orders the supplies. If a practice normally has a medical assistant or nurse order supplies, that task should be rotated among all of the nurses or medical assistants. This rotation of duties helps to prevent inappropriate relationships between vendors and employees. In cases of collusion among the employees and a salesperson, rotation of duties can often expose these inappropriate relationships.

Finally, medical groups should set and enforce limits on the dollar volume that employees at various levels can commit to on behalf of the practice. This policy ensures that oversight is provided on a progressive basis. For example, a practice could adopt a policy that sets purchasing limits as shown in Exhibit 3.

These limits could be adjusted based on the size of the practice.

Recommendation summary:

- Develop policies and procedures for ordering, such as using ordering calendars or an inventory alert system;
- Rotate the ordering responsibility among practice employees; and
- Enforce ordering policies that limit the dollar amount of goods and services that employees can order without additional approval.

EXHIBIT 3

Sample Purchasing Limits for a Medical Practice

Commitment Level	Authorized Employee
$500	Medical assistant or nurse
$1,000	Clinic or office manager
$2,500	Practice administrator or CEO
$5,000	Physician president or managing physician
$10,000	Board of directors
Over $10,000	Shareholders

6. Follow Up and Schedule the Order

Following up on a supply order is the routine tracking of the order to ensure that the goods are delivered when needed. In the past, follow-up was done exclusively by telephone, but today supply chain and delivery systems make it easy to track orders online.

In identifying possible vendors, it is important to get references on the delivery reliability of the vendor. If a vendor has problems delivering as scheduled, the vendor should be willing to expedite a shipment at no additional cost. If a vendor is chronically late in its deliveries, that vendor should be excluded from future bidding. Medical groups must develop systems to follow up on the timely delivery of orders.

Expediting is applying pressure to a vendor or supplier to meet an accelerated delivery schedule or speed up the delivery of a late order. Expediting is usually done by telephone and sometimes requires going to the sales manager. Practices should have a system in place to elevate the expediting process when necessary.

Recommendation summary:

- Screen vendors based on delivery reliability;

- Implement a routine follow-up system; and
- Expedite orders that are late and do not be afraid to ask the vendor to use a more expensive shipping method if the vendor does not deliver on time through its normal channels.

7. Receive, Inspect, and Store the Goods

A formal receiving process is important to confirm that the placed order has arrived in good condition and with the correct quantity. The receiving process also directs the goods to the destination where they will be used or stored and ensures that the proper receiving documentation is reviewed, approved, and forwarded. Practices should plan storage close to where the goods and supplies are to be used.

If possible, to strengthen internal controls, the order should be received and checked by someone who was not responsible for placing the order. It is also important to make sure the quantity received is correct, because distributors will sometimes make partial shipments when the distributor is running low on stock. Occasionally, an order will be shorted but billed as a full order.

Recommendation summary:

- Establish a process for receiving and checking goods delivered;
- Store the goods as close to the user site as possible;
- Have the order received and checked by someone other than the individual who placed the order; and
- Always double check the quantity received.

8. Approve the Invoice

The next step in the purchasing process is to approve the invoice. The invoice approval process can vary according to the practice. Sometimes the invoice is sent to the user department where the original purchase was made. When this happens, the using department will match the invoice with the receiving documents to make sure the goods that have been billed have been received and accepted; also, the using department manager will approve the invoice and forward the complete set of paperwork to the practice's accounting department.

In other cases, the invoices are mailed to the accounting department, where they are matched with the receiving documents and then paid. Whichever method is implemented, it is important that invoices be paid only after approving the paperwork that documents that the goods or services were received in good condition.

If there are discrepancies between the invoice and receiving documentation, it is often best to have the accounting department, who is independent of the ordering and receiving function, follow up on the discrepancy.

Recommendation summary:

- Approve invoices in the ordering department or the accounting department; and
- Have the accounting department follow up on any discrepancies.

9. Pay the Supplier

Once the goods and services have been received and checked, the receiving documents matched with the invoices, and all discrepancies resolved, the vendor invoices should be paid as promised. Normally vendors request payment within 30 days of the invoice, and these requests should be honored if the vendors or distributors have provided goods or services as ordered.

Vendors sometimes provide discounts for early payment of their invoices. If vendors offer these discounts to your practice, it is usually cost-effective to take advantage of it.

Some practices try to conserve their cash or maximize their investment earnings by delaying vendor payments for 60 or even 90 days. Unless there is a good reason to delay such payments, like a new piece of equipment not functioning properly, it is usually best to pay vendors promptly. If a practice needs special treatment from a vendor, that vendor is much more likely to grant the practice's request if the practice has paid the vendor on time.

Vendor payments should be entered into the practice's accounts payable system in such a way to prevent the inadvertent duplicate payment of invoices. Once paid, the invoices should be cancelled or otherwise clearly marked as paid.

Recommendation summary:

- Pay vendors promptly unless there is a problem with the goods or services;
- Cancel invoices or mark them clearly as paid to prevent duplicate payments; and
- Implement accounting system safeguards to prevent the same invoice number from being paid a second time.

10. Use Goods and Services

The final step in the purchasing process is to use the goods and services that have been ordered. This step entails removing goods from inventory and using them in the practice's clinical or business process. When inventory is depleted to a certain level, the purchasing cycle is begun again. For recurring purchases, the cycle goes from step 10 to step 5, which is reordering. If new items are needed, the practice will follow steps 1 through 4. Periodically, a practice should solicit new vendor bids for goods and services, as noted in step 4.

Group Purchasing Organizations

GPOs are organizations that negotiate for the purchase of medical goods and services on behalf of their members, which include hospitals, nursing homes, medical practices, and other provider organizations. Hospitals have been using GPOs for several years, and today more and more medical practices are taking advantage of the buying power and economies of scale that GPOs can provide.

EXHIBIT 4

GPO Purchasing Volume

Ranked by 2005 purchasing volume ($ in millions)[18]

Organization	Location	2005 Volume
Premier Purchasing Partners	Charlotte, NC	$27,397
Novation	Irving, TX	$25,400
MedAssets	Alpharetta, GA	$12,000
HealthTrust Purchasing Group	Brentwood, TN	$7,500
Broadlane	Dallas, TX	$6,579
Amerinet	St. Louis, MO	$6,350
Consorta	Schaumburg, IL	$4,240
GNYHA Ventures	New York, NY	$3,390
HealthCare Purchasing Partners Int'l.	Irving, TX	$2,500
Innovatix	New York, NY	$2,000

Some GPOs have staff that can assist practices in developing and refining their purchasing process. A listing of the major GPOs and 2005 purchasing volume is shown in Exhibit 4.

If a practice is not part of a GPO, it should consider joining one. GPO membership is often available at no cost through many trade associations (including MGMA) or through the medical staff affiliation of a group's physicians.

Summary

The purchasing cycle in a medical practice is a critical business function. The purchasing function not only ensures that a practice has the right goods and services at the right time to meet the needs of its patients, providers, and staff, but it also ensures that these goods and services are available at the best price. Medical practice employees involved in the purchasing function are usually not well prepared or trained to deal with sales professionals of medical suppliers. In most practices, the purchasing function is at risk for inefficiency in procurement as well as fraud. Fortunately, practices can take simple and practical steps to strengthen their purchasing function and protect itself against irregularities and fraud.

Chapter 3 Managing the Organization's Facilities

THE DESIGN, construction, maintenance, and appearance of a practice's offices are critical to the efficiency of the practice. As with any business or place of public accommodation, the outward appearance of a facility sets a foundation for the client/patient's expectation of the level and quality of service that will be provided. Facilities that are dark with threadbare carpeting and dingy walls will be perceived by clients as providing second-rate service; facilities that are well lit, clean, and neat will be perceived as providing a much higher level of service.

The design or layout of a facility, although normally transparent to the patient, will have far-reaching effects on the efficiency of the physicians and staff. Clinical areas that are designed to allow easy access to the supplies and support services that may be required during the course of the day will enable physicians and staff to be more productive and effective. Failure to be attentive to proper office design may result in a variety of problems, including physicians and staff becoming overtired because of excessive walking and the duplication of expensive supply inventories within examination rooms in an effort to reduce these walking demands.

When the opportunity exists to either design a new facilities plan, or significantly renovate an existing space, it is best to utilize the expertise of an architect who is well versed and experienced in the design and construction of medical office space. In designing or renovating facilities, applicable building codes and regulations have to be integrated. These issues, which span local, state, and federal agencies, create a range of structural requirements that require compliance to ensure a safe environment. In most instances, local building codes will provide the requirements for construction issues, including wiring and plumbing standards; width of corridors; and heating, ventilation, and air conditioning minimums. Sufficient insulation between rooms and noise-dampening materials should also be used in construction to help ensure patient privacy.

Federal guidelines that require compliance are primarily represented by the regulations of the Americans with Disabilities Act of 1990 (ADA) and the Occupational Safety and Health Administration (OSHA). The primary goal of the ADA, as it applies to facilities, is to ensure that individuals with disabilities have safe and easy access to and can maneuver within a place of public accommodation. To comply within the parameters of the ADA, a practice needs to address physical design features such as ensuring that doors are wide enough to allow for the passage of a wheelchair, having restroom facilities available that can be easily used by the disabled, and providing adequate designated handicapped parking. In cases where the physical space is not owned by the practice, meeting these expectations will be the responsibility of building management.

The safety of staff, patients, and visitors is addressed through adherence to the regulations set forth by OSHA. These safety issues include the proper maintenance, use, and storage of equipment, or addressing any hazardous situation, such as loose extension cords and boxes that are stacked too high. Other safety issues concern access to proper fire prevention equipment and the installation of security alarms and/or cameras, where appropriate. In addition to setting forth guidelines and regulations to ensure the safety of patients, visitors, and staff, OSHA regulations require the organization to maintain logs and information on all accidents and injuries that occur on the premises. Through these reports, issues affecting the safety and well-being of everyone are maintained.

When designing or renovating a facility, attentiveness to small details that enable a facility to be both efficient and attractive are important. Patients and visitors coming to the facility require appropriate signage to assist them in reaching the correct office or location within the practice. Adequate signage is also important to assist new employees in becoming familiar with the office and building layout. Appropriate color schemes for walls, flooring, and furniture are helpful in maintaining a relaxing and inviting environment for patients who might otherwise be stressful and anxious.

In addition to the design of the clinical areas, attention should be paid to the business areas of the practice, which patients never see, including billing, scheduling, medical records, accounting, human resources, and storage. Failure to design these areas properly and to provide for sufficient storage space will have a direct negative impact on the ability of the support staff to adequately complete their job assignments.

No matter how well a facility is designed and decorated, though, without proper preventive maintenance, the significant investment that is made in creating the facility will soon lose its value. Preventive maintenance includes such day-to-day issues as trash removal, vacuuming, dusting, and mopping. In addition, other maintenance items need to be scheduled on a regular basis, including window washing, touch-up painting, replacement of dim or burned-out bulbs, and minor cosmetic repairs of furniture and equipment. Patients are very quick to identify housekeeping issues and equate them to the quality of the medical services provided. Although patients may not comment when facilities are clean and well maintained, they do notice (and comment) when their expectations are not met, and they apply their observations to determining the professionalism and quality of the physicians of the practice.

The concept of facility design and maintenance goes beyond the confines of the four walls of the practice's office; attention should also be paid to ensuring that adequate, safe parking is available and that the grounds surrounding the building are properly maintained and landscaped. The building should appear inviting, without dark corridors or foreboding entranceways. Patients have choices of where to obtain their medical services, and it is incumbent upon the practice to provide a safe and welcoming environment.

Chapter 4

Utilizing Experts and Business Partners

THE BENEFITS OF ALLIANCES are undeniable. According to Ernst and Young, organizations that form successful alliances can earn more than 20 percent of their revenues in such relationships.[19] In fact, this number has grown and continues to increase. Research indicates that some organizations expect their alliances to contribute 35 percent of their revenues in the future, up from 21 percent in 1998 and 15 percent in 1995.[20]

An alliance is a cooperative arrangement between two or more physician groups that allows these organizations to combine in a common effort to gain or maintain competitive advantage. The mere formation of an alliance does not guarantee success, but rather requires mutual participation of all parties, a viable business concept, and a realistic strategy to implementing that idea.[21]

Alliances should be strategic in nature rather than a short-term solution to an immediate problem. Medical practice executives need to look past short-term gains and focus on building long-term goals for alliances and partnerships.

Key Issues in Alliances

A number of key questions should be considered when forming an alliance, including:

- What is the purpose of the alliance?
- What partner or partners should be selected?
- What is the structure of the alliance?
- What are the roles and responsibilities of the parties involved?
- What are the risks involved?
- What is the duration of the alliance?

Purpose of the Alliance

Prior to considering an alliance, a clearly defined purpose has to be established. Without a clear vision, organizations will waste time, money, and energy entering into alliances and partnerships that do not meet their organization's needs.

The primary motivation for many health care organizations to engage in alliances and partnerships is due to the conflicting demands of cost-containment, delivering high-quality care, and expanding access to services. Alliances and partnerships are the vehicles that enable medical group practices that do not possess the necessary resources individually to combine resources with other organizations to gain competitive advantage in the health care marketplace.[22]

Competitive advantage typically serves two purposes: (1) reduce dependence, and (2) improve organizational capacity. Ways in which organizations reduce dependence can be achieved through vertical integration, by which individual practices provide complementary services, thereby expanding access to a wider variety of services for their patients. By forming alliances, an individual organization is able to gain access to technology, expertise, labor, and possibly even capital, thus expanding its capacity. Another way practices can increase organizational capacity is by forming alliances to share risk, so that individual organizations can enter new markets without having to bear all the financial risk of uncertain conditions inherent in new ventures. Alliances also help individual organizations to overcome regulatory barriers, increase organizational flexibility, improve access to technological innovations, and achieve efficiency through economies of scale.[23]

Partner Selection

It is critical to select alliance partners that leverage one another's strengths. Alliances are not a quick fix for all of an organization's deficiencies. Alliances are similar to relationships – each person has a distinct identity and personality. Alliances, like relationships, unite unique parties to work together for a common cause. Just like relationships, however, there are negatives associated with alliances as well. Alliances bring organizations' employees together, with any cultural differences they may have. For instance, one organization may possess formal, clear management structures, while the other operates informally and forms only ad hoc arrangements. To be successful, alliance partners must share compatible, but not necessarily identical, cultures and missions or the alliance will fail.

Differences can be a source of conflict, and they should be anticipated. Alliance partners need to keep their common interests in mind at all times. The following tips can help to resolve most conflicts that arise in alliances: (1) clarify the issue; (2) have each organization present its point of view; (3) seek to understand each partner's point of view; (4) discuss differences that arise; and (5) always agree to solve the problem collaboratively.[24]

It is the medical practice executive's role to watch for these warning signs of conflict and in a productive way to resolve it.[25] Warning signs that conflict is imminent include: (1) an issue repeatedly arises, (2) individual(s) choose not to listen during meetings and discussions, and (3) individuals seem to avoid one another. Practice executives should be proactive to overcome possible shortcomings before they become a major issue.

This initial step in establishing an alliance requires screening and selecting potential partners. In order to do so, it is critical first to understand the practice's own objectives, its capabilities, and its resources or lack thereof. Without a full understanding and accounting for all alliance strategy issues internally, decisions about whom to partner with will be uninformed.[26]

Ideal candidates for alliances will have compatible objectives, complementary resources and skills, an organizational fit in terms of culture and processes, and a willingness to ally with each other. Although collecting this information can be difficult and time consuming, the payoff for understanding a potential partner's objectives, financials, resources, skills, processes, and culture can be priceless.[27] It is also important to consult with each potential practice's legal counsel to understand the ramifications of aligning with a particular organization.

Choosing the Appropriate Structure

When considering alliances, many models are available to strengthen a practice's competitive position. Depending on the level of integration or degree of cooperation required, organizations can pick from any of the following types of affiliations. In general, this list begins with the least integrated and finishes with the most complex.

Network Affiliation

Network affiliations are the least-integrated type of alliance and function as a club with a general purpose. They provide a useful avenue for supportive dialogue, communication, and commiseration; however, they are not functional for contracting or for implementation activities.[28]

Joint Ventures

Joint ventures are typically formed for a well-defined goal that is typically focused on capital projects. According to Ginter, Swayne, and Duncan, "a joint venture is the combination of the resources of two or more separate organizations to accomplish a designated task.... When projects get too large, technology too expensive, or the costs of failure too high for a single organization, joint ventures are often used."[29] The term "joint venture" applies to a wide range of interorganizational arrangements and frequently concerns physician-related ventures.

Joint ventures can provide medical practices with a competitive strategy, typically in an undeveloped or underdeveloped market, moving more directly from existing providers to a more convenient alternative for a targeted population. One advantage of joint ventures is that they can be quickly formed to take advantage of fast-moving opportunities. They also allow organizations otherwise constrained by resources and capabilities to effectively pursue opportunities together.[30]

As in all the models of alliances, joint ventures can be difficult because of the clash of culture and compatibility between organizations. Allied organizations need to be on the same page, but need not abandon their identity or their organizational culture to collaborate successfully. To avoid casualties from the culture clash, explicit mechanisms need to be developed to identify and manage these challenges.[31]

Independent Provider Associations and Provider Organizations

Independent provider associations (IPAs) and provider organizations (POs) are typically formed to organize independent medical group practices for the purpose of contracting with health maintenance organizations and purchasing supplies or other services. The main difference between IPAs and POs is that IPAs typically are affiliated with a hospital.[32]

One primary advantage of IPAs is that they offer a variety of physician choices to their members. They also tend to be more acceptable to managed care organizations (MCOs) than other, less traditional integrated delivery system models. Another reason IPAs are attractive is that they require much less capital to start and maintain as opposed to other models available.[33]

IPAs are not without disadvantages, though. For example, because IPAs are one of the least-integrated forms of alliances, they do not offer the opportunity to leverage resources and achieve economies of scale that more integrated forms offer. In addition, management of this loose type of alliance structure can be challenging because individual physician practices maintain their independence in an IPA. This issue grows as more practices enter the IPA.[34]

Physician/Hospital Organizations

Physician/Hospital Organizations (PHOs) involve physicians and hospitals whereby they become partners in the delivery of health care. Exclusivity is an issue because most PHOs contain a selection process to qualify the doctors involved. The ownership arrangements of PHOs vary widely; however, most strive to provide physicians and hospitals an equal voice and ownership. In most PHOs, the hospital organization may supply the most capital; however, board composition does not typically reflect this equity position.[35]

PHOs have the advantage of being inexpensive to form and maintain. They are also desirable to many group practices because they maintain group autonomy and, thus, are nonthreatening. One of the biggest advantages that PHOs provide is the ability to negotiate on behalf of their membership. Additionally, they provide an opportunity for greater integration between a hospital and its medical staff.[36]

Along with these advantages come several disadvantages, including the unpredictable nature of these affiliations. Because these affiliations are loose, they are often ineffective and do not provide partners with economies of scale or improvement in contracting ability. In fact, MCOs often view PHOs as a barrier to effective communication with individual practitioners, thus decreasing the effectiveness of utilization of management activities.[37] MCOs often choose to deal directly with individual physicians because they desire the right to select providers themselves.

Management Services Organizations

Management services organizations (MSOs) are typically formed to provide management services and administrative systems to one or more medical group practices. MSOs are normally based on one or more health care organizations. For example, MSOs may conduct billing, marketing, or perhaps the human resource functions for its members. Each medical practice remains a separate entity and chooses whether to use the services that the MSO offers. In addition to providing the above services, many MSOs purchase the assets of the physicians' practice.[38]

MSOs are more closely aligned with the hospital as compared to PHOs. MSOs provide their members the economies of scale and also the advantage of sharing data regarding practice behavior, which can help to increase the effectiveness of individual practices.[39]

Similar to the PHO, physicians in an MSO remain independent contractors and thus maintain the ability to change allegiances, a downside to this type of affiliation. This point may also be considered an advantage, though, especially from the physician's viewpoint. Another disadvantage is the hospital mind-set, in which physician practices are viewed as another hospital department, negatively impacting the practice's performance.[40]

Group Practice Without Walls

Group practice without walls (GPWWs) are not true alliances because individual groups or sites can continue to manage themselves. GPWWs offer a higher level of integration of physician services and do not require the participation of a hospital organization. Most GPWWs are formed to address antitrust or hazards of the Stark self-referral law. In fact, a GPWW is a legal merging of all assets of the physician practice, which is different than the acquisition of tangible assets, as in the MSO.[41]

An advantage of this type of affiliation is that each site maintains its independence, and thus is easy to manage and does not have to sacrifice much autonomy; however, GPWWs help to present a united front to MCOs because they have the legal ability to negotiate and commit resources on behalf of their members. Because of the increased level of integration, GPWWs are able to achieve a moderate level of economies of scale. Examples may include shared billing, group purchasing, contracting for human resources, and payroll. Because the financial performances of its members are dependent upon one another, GPWWs are able to exert pressure and influence the practice behavior of their members.[42]

Perhaps the primary disadvantage associated with GPWWs is the fact that individual medical practices are still independent. This can present a managerial challenge to align incentives, even though fiscal performance in a GPWW is dependent on one another. Another disadvantage that is linked to the independence of the physician practices is that the overall leadership is typically weaker than that found in the medical groups that form the GPWW.[43]

Single-Specialty Group Practices

Single-specialty group practices include only physicians of the same specialty and provide a significant level of integration. Single-specialty groups share a common billing number, fee schedule, benefits package, and a formal governance structure.

Multispecialty Group Practices

Multispecialty group practices are practices that include multiple specialties and disciplines. Multispecialty group practices must be formed to ensure that the group includes the right mix of specialties and the appropriate proportions to allow for a mutually beneficial existence.[44]

Multispecialty group practices are advantageous because they can accept capitation, are able to leverage economies of scale, offer an environment conducive for the exchange of ideas between physicians, and are attractive to MCOs. Despite these advantages, they have the potential to threaten the existing autonomy of individual specialties and consequently can be functionally challenging to manage.[45]

Due Diligence Process

To minimize exposure to risk when embarking on a strategic alliance or partnership, it is critical to conduct due diligence to ensure that the proposed venture is a prudent decision. Due diligence entails collecting information and data in order to assess the feasibility of a particular venture so that a decision is reached only after considering all prudent viewpoints. Due diligence should take place on numerous fronts, including recruiting, membership in a strategic alliance, considering managed care contracts, adopting new technology, marketing campaigns, and compensation of employees. Due diligence is a complex activity, especially in light of considering strategic alliances. Thus, a knowledgeable health care attorney should be consulted when considering opportunities and drafting essential legal documents.[46]

Recruiting

Ensuring the effective and successful recruitment of personnel, including physicians, is a critical responsibility of the medical practice executive. Due diligence should be conducted to ensure that personnel are qualified and that they fit the culture of the organization. Medical practice executives should understand the marketplace prior to conducting a search process so they can respond to candidates' questions, be familiar with the most effective sources for personnel, set clear expectations about the time frame needed for the search, and understand the financial implications of attracting and hiring staff.[47]

In addition, medical practices need to present an appealing practice environment in order to attract quality personnel. Prospective employees are not only interested in pleasant surroundings, they are also concerned with the financial stability, up-to-date technology, and attractive schedules and policies. By ensuring that these concerns are addressed, medical practice executives will be more successful in selling the organization to prospective employees and reduce failure and future turnover.[48]

Due diligence is especially critical when recruiting physicians to join the medical practice. If due diligence is not practiced, effective personnel will not be attracted or retained, and thus the organization will likely perform poorly or fail.

Strategic Alliances

Due diligence is a crucial part of the alliance process. Thus, whenever feasible, a more comprehensive due diligence investigation should be undertaken when considering whether to partner with a particular organization. However, because of the costly and time-consuming nature of the process, it is not always feasible to investigate every detail of a potential strategic alliance. Thus, when considering smaller alliances and transactions, too much due diligence can kill the transaction.[49]

Key questions to assist in the due diligence of a potential strategic alliance include the following:

- What in the alliance is important to your medical group practice? What isn't?
- Which problems will be costly? Which ones will be minor?
- Where are you likely to find problems? Where are you unlikely to find problems?
- What type of transaction are you expecting? How large or small is the transaction? How complex? What will the due diligence investigation cost in time and money?
- What is the risk to your medical group practice if the unexpected causes the transaction to go bad?
- How much time do you have? What do you have to lose by delay? What does the potential partner have to lose? How important to your medical practice is the alliance? How important is your practice to the potential partners?[50]

Additionally, more specific questions can be asked to further clarify whether a potential merger is a prudent move. For instance:

- What is the organization's public image? Have there been any tensions between the community and the organization?
- Are there any pending lawsuits against the organization?
- Does the organization have a good reputation?
- How long has the organization been in business?
- Is the organization financially stable?[51]

Managed Care Contracts

When considering partnerships and strategic alliances, it is critical to review all managed care contracts – both old and new. Frequently, new alliances may change the structure of current contracts, particularly the reimbursement mechanisms for physicians. Thus, it is important to review and decide whether to continue the contracts in the present form or make changes. Another important consideration regarding managed care contracting is that the structure of the proposed partnership or alliance may actually make renegotiating contracts more favorable for reimbursement levels.[52]

Technology

The technological know-how of each partner involved in a potential alliance must also be considered because of the costly nature of technology. For instance, if the medical practice is currently using a paper-based medical records system, it may be inordinately expensive to convert to electronic health records to facilitate the alliance. Often, the expense of adopting new technology may outweigh the benefits of the potential partnership.

Marketing

The power of marketing cannot be overlooked. A carefully constructed marketing campaign can assist a new partnership or alliance in rapidly succeeding, especially in generating cash flow. Thus, medical practice executives need to carefully align marketing to showcase their new organizational form to make the practice's current patients, future patients, and the medical community aware of its existence to retain or expand its current client base.[53]

Physician Compensation

Physician compensation must be carefully evaluated prior to considering potential partnerships and alliances. Conflict can arise when a medical practice whose physicians are dependent on a salary compensation structure attempt to partner or align with a practice whose physicians have an ownership approach to compensation. Another area to consider is that of benefits packages, as physicians in integrated organizations typically receive more generous packages than a new group can offer, thus potentially contributing to discord.[54]

Roles and Responsibilities

Successful alliances require well-defined processes to address key issues in alliance formation, implementation, and operation; thus, it is necessary to structure and negotiate agreement with each partner. The strategic objectives of the alliance should be evaluated and aligned to increase the probability of success. It is at this stage that staffing decisions should be considered, with all partners striving for a reasonable share of control that facilitates equitable involvement from all sides. Because alliances are a long-term venture, it is advisable to commit the best personnel who are striving for long-term placement; otherwise, high turnover can doom the alliance before it gets started. Alliance relationships take time to build and gain trust; thus frequently changing alliance personnel can disrupt the process.[55] Knowledge about the practice's capabilities is particularly important for defining work roles and supporting the requirements of current and future partners.[56]

At the outset of the partnership, alliance partners should collaboratively set goals and measure performance parameters that are quantifiable. These goals and measures should be congruent with the alliance's primary objectives. Additionally, alliance partners should address governance issues and develop an operating framework built around the clearly defined roles and expectations of each partner. Without resolving these critical issues, the success of the alliance may be in jeopardy.

Risks

Risk is a significant factor in the formation of alliances because strategic decision making is ultimately concerned with assessing odds for success.[57] One of the primary advantages of joining an alliance is to control uncertainty and exposure to risk. Risk can be defined as unanticipated or negative variation, typically associated with negative outcomes. Risk sharing or risk controlling is a key justification for joining strategic alliances.[58]

Two types of risks are generally associated with alliances: (1) relational risk, or the probability that one or more partners does not comply with the rules governing the alliance; and (2) performance risk, which refers to the probability that the intended strategic goals of the alliance may not be achieved despite diligent cooperation among the partners.[59]

Duration

As with strategic plans, alliances should be reviewed and evaluated on an annual basis to estimate their effectiveness and worth – similar to how a portfolio of investments should be viewed. Using this approach allows the organizations to manage, review, and evaluate alliances as an aggregate business, and it permits the organization to evaluate current resource allocations with a focus on identifying how alliance concentrations contribute to possible duplication or gaps.[60]

While conducting an ongoing evaluation, it is important for the organization to develop an effective working environment with all partners to facilitate the completion of the actual work. It is critical to include performance measures combined with feedback from alliance partners to assess the progress of the alliance.

If an alliance is not functioning as intended and is not salvageable, it is appropriate to end the association. Often, this is due to a change in market conditions, and no one is to blame for the ending of the alliance. Regardless of the reason for the termination of the alliance, it is important for the practice to maintain a positive relationship with the former partners, as new opportunities for collaboration may present themselves in the future.[61]

Managing Partnerships and Strategic Alliances

Management of alliances should be approached in a fashion similar to how organizations should be managed. As in all organizations, medical practice executives should continually acknowledge and actively monitor the concerns of all legitimate stakeholders and shareholders, and should take their interests into consideration when making operational decisions. A stakeholder is anyone who has an investment in the success of the organization, including physicians, administrators, patients, vendors, and the community. Shareowners have a special status among stakeholders in that the potential gain or loss from their involvement with the corporation is determined by the organization's profit margin.[62]

Practice executives should maintain open lines of communication with stakeholders about their respective concerns and contributions, and about the risks that they assume due to their involvement with the corporation.[63] The more open managers can be about critical decisions and their consequences, and the more clearly managers understand and appreciate the perspectives and concerns of affected parties, the more likely it is that problematic situations can be satisfactorily resolved. Open communication and dialogue are, in themselves, stakeholder benefits, quite apart from their content or the conclusions.[64]

By virtue of being part of an alliance, organizations lose some freedom to make decisions without concern for alliance partners. The medical practice executive should be sensitive to the concerns and capabilities of the other alliance stakeholders. To maintain the survival of the alliance, the interdependence of efforts among the alliance partners must be recognized. All attempts should be made to achieve a fair distribution of rewards and burdens in the alliance, and at the same time to account for each organization's vulnerabilities.[65]

A commitment to engage in dialogue, however, does not constitute a commitment to collective decision making. There are obvious limits to the amount and content of information (particularly information about strategic options under consideration) that can be appropriately shared with particular stakeholder groups.

Practice executives should acknowledge that conflict is an inevitable part of alliances, as it is with all interactions with people. In the interests of all parties involved, any conflicts should be handled openly and fairly, and, where necessary, by third-party review. Maintaining fairness and openness will guarantee that all parties will act responsibly and not threaten the existence of the alliance.[66]

Summary

An appreciation of alliances can assist medical practice executives in understanding the resources and dedication necessary to establish such partnerships. Alliances enable medical practices to strategically position themselves and gain competitive advantage to survive in today's turbulent health care market.

Chapter 5

Directing the Marketing and Communication Plans

If the circus is coming to town and you paint a sign saying, "Circus is coming to Fairgrounds Sunday," that's Advertising. If you put the sign on the back of an elephant and walk him through town, that's a Promotion. If the elephant walks through the Mayor's flower bed, that's Publicity. If you can get the Mayor to laugh about it, that's Public Relations. And, if you planned the whole thing, that's Marketing!

– Author Unknown

IN GENERAL, marketing activities are all those activities associated with identifying the particular wants and needs of a target market of customers, and then going about satisfying those customers better than the competition does. This involves doing market research on customers, analyzing their needs, and then making strategic decisions about product design, pricing, promotion, and distribution. This view is consistent with the following definition of marketing found in a popular marketing textbook: "Marketing is the process of planning and executing the conception, pricing, promotion, and distribution of ideas, goods, services, organizations, and events to create and maintain relationships that will satisfy individual and organizational objectives."[67]

Components of a Marketing Plan

To accomplish the "marketing" tasks identified in these definitions, a marketing plan similar to the strategic and business plans needs to be developed. This marketing plan follows a framework similar to those of the other plans: executive summary, situational analysis, marketing objectives, marketing strategies, and so on.

Executive Summary

The executive summary of the practice's marketing plan should address the following key elements:

- What are the dominant issues discovered in the practice's situational analysis?
- What are the key objectives the practice seeks to achieve – in the shortest possible form?
- What, in one or two sentences, is the practice's marketing strategy to achieve those objectives?
- What other concepts unique to the practice should be addressed?

Answers to these questions comprise the body of the marketing plan; therefore, the executive summary cannot be written until the plan has been completed. It will then serve as the "snapshot" of what the practice aims to accomplish with regard to strategic marketing.

Situational Analysis

The situational analysis investigates the macro- and microenvironment in a manner similar to the strategic plan. In fact, the same tool – the SWOT (strengths, weaknesses, opportunities, and threats)analysis – can be used in this stage of the marketing plan process. The practice should review its strategic plan's SWOT and then consider each of the SWOT's components from a consumer and market viewpoint: its external threats and opportunities, its internal strengths and weaknesses, including key success factors in the health care industry, and the practice's sustainable competitive advantage. Along with the strategic plan's SWOT analysis, a two-by-two matrix can be created to identify specific focus areas for the marketing plan: the macroenvironment, the internal practice environment, market analyses, and consumer analyses (see Exhibit 5).

Macroenvironmental analysis refers to continuous structured data collection and processing on a broad range of environmental factors, such as the economy, the governmental and legal environments, technology, and social culture. This allows the practice to

EXHIBIT 5

Marketing Plan Situational Analysis Two-by-Two Matrix

Macroenvironment	Market Analysis
What does your practice do well? ▪ Innovative leadership ▪ Good reputation	*Where are the opportunities for your practice?* ▪ Untapped market for new procedure ▪ Hiring new physician in practice ▪ Need for geriatric care in community
Consumer Analysis	**Internal Practice Analysis**
What part of your practice needs improvement? ▪ High nurse turnover ▪ Location of practice ▪ Retiring physician ▪ Providing geriatric care	*What is happening in your area that could threaten your practice?* ▪ New regulation ▪ Growing elderly population

act quickly, take advantage of opportunities before competitors do, and respond to environmental threats before significant damage is done. Scanning these macroenvironmental variables for threats and opportunities requires that each issue be rated on two dimensions: (1) its potential impact on the practice, and (2) its likelihood of occurrence. Weighing its potential impact by its likelihood of occurrence provides an indication of its importance to the practice.

The microenvironmental, or internal, analysis seeks to uncover the resources of the practice that apply or can be applied to marketing efforts. These resources include money, time, people, and skills. What internal resources does the practice have that are underexploited? Finding these resources internally as opposed to having to seek them externally will provide countless benefits to the practice. Along with identification of resources, the practice's vision, mission, and goals (in particular, long-term goals/objectives, marketing goals/objectives, and financial goals/objectives) should be reviewed, and the culture of the practice should be considered. Each of these areas will have an impact on the marketing strategy of the practice.

A consumer analysis explores the demographic makeup of the practice's consumer base, but also delves a bit deeper into the consumers' purchasing and decision-making behaviors, their motivations and expectations, and loyalty segments. Who are the practice's current consumers? What brought them to the practice in the first place?

The final piece of the situational analysis is the market analysis. In the market analysis, the medical practice defines its market; identifies its market size and industry market trends; evaluates the market segmentation and strategic groups; and studies the competition's strengths, weaknesses, and market share. A tool often used in completing these tasks is Michael Porter's Five Forces Analysis,[68] which allows a systematic and structured analysis of market structure and competitive situation. The five forces consist of those forces close to a company that affect its ability to serve its customers and make a profit.

Four of the forces – the bargaining power of consumers, the bargaining power of suppliers, the threat of new entrants, and the threat of substitute products – combine with other variables to influence

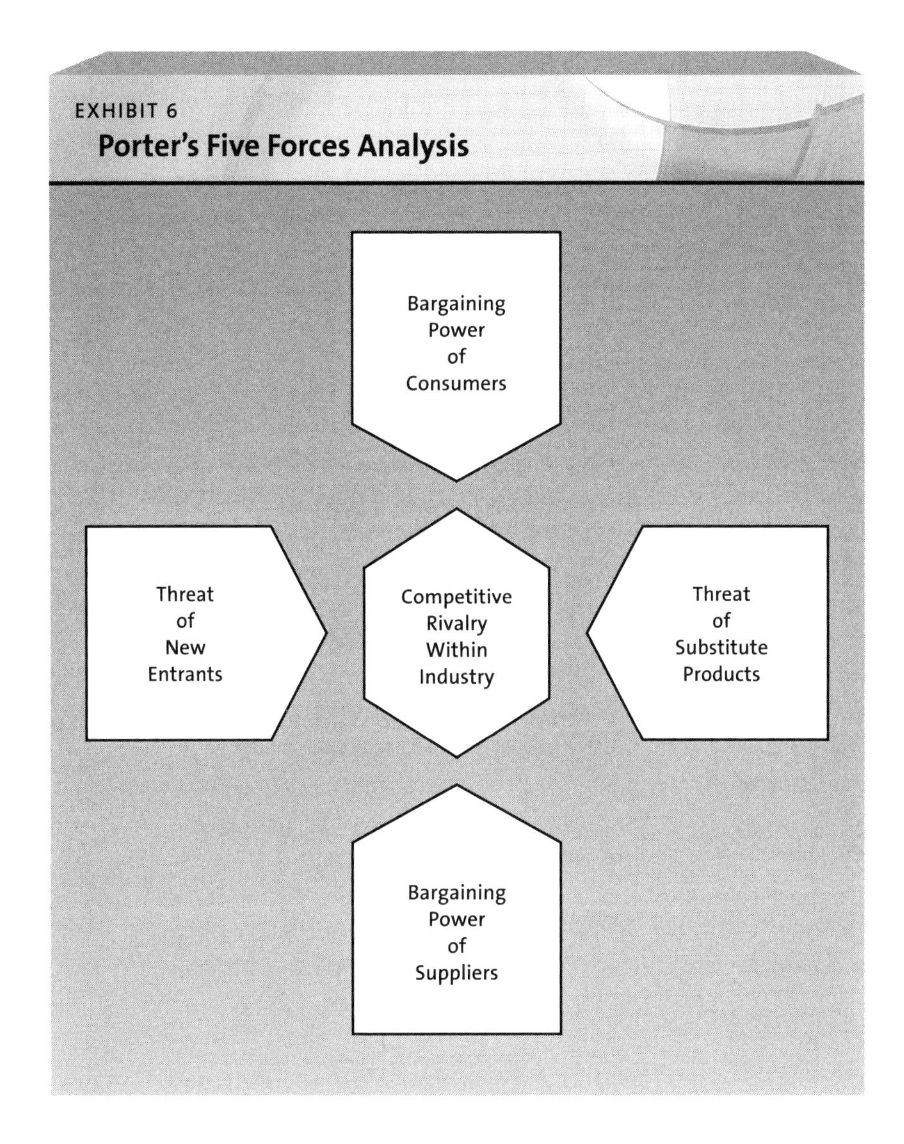

a fifth force, the level of competition in an industry. A change in any of the forces normally requires a practice to reassess the marketplace. Exhibit 6 illustrates Porter's Five Forces Analysis.

The bargaining power of customers determines how much pressure on margins and volumes customers can impose. For example, customers will have high bargaining power when the ability to switch to an alternative product (e.g., a new prescription plan) is relatively simple and is not related to high costs, or when the customers have low margins and are price sensitive (e.g., a small practice with few employees on a plan, but still needing a good price). The bargaining power of suppliers is similar. The term "suppliers" comprises all sources for inputs that are needed in order to provide goods or services. In such situations, the buying industry often faces high pressure on margins from its suppliers. The relationship to powerful suppliers can potentially reduce strategic options for the practice.

When there is a threat of new entrants in the community that will compete with the practice, changes may occur in the major determinants of the market environment (e.g., market shares, prices, patient and staff loyalty) at any time. Remember that there is always a latent pressure for reaction and adjustment for existing competitors in the health care industry. A threat from substitutes exists if there are alternative products or services, or complementary products or services, with lower prices and/or higher quality that can be used for the same purpose. These competitors could potentially attract a significant proportion of market volume and consequently reduce the potential sales volume. Competitive rivalry within the industry derives the intensity of competition among existing practices. High competitive pressure results in pressure on prices, margins, and profitability for every single company in the industry.

After the analysis of the current and potential future state of the five forces, the practice can search for options to influence these forces in its favor, thereby reducing the competitive forces' power.

Marketing Research

Marketing research is the next major task undertaken in the marketing plan process. The American Marketing Association defines marketing research as:

> ...the function that links the consumer, customer, and public to the marketer through information – information used to identify and define marketing opportunities and problems; generate, refine, and evaluate marketing actions; monitor marketing per-

formance; and improve understanding of marketing as a process. Market research specifies the information required to address these issues, designs the method for collecting information, manages and implements the data collection process, analyzes the results, and communicates the findings and their implications.[69]

The aim of marketing research is to find out the who, what, when, and where with regard to the practice's customers and services: Who are the customers? What services do they want? When do they want these services provided? Where do they want these services provided? Answers to these questions can reveal problems with current services as well as potential trends for the future. In addition to identifying the practice's customers and their preferences, market research should assist the practice in determining its market share and the effectiveness of its advertising and promotions.

Three general sources of market data can be gathered: (1) data already available externally (e.g., from the chamber of commerce, business coalitions, state trade organizations, and the U.S. Census Bureau); (2) data readily available internally (e.g., from employees, current customers, and company records and files); and (3) data that can be collected by and/or for the practice (e.g., through surveys, interviews, evaluation/response cards, customer feedback, and observations of competition). The practice executive should determine what form of market research will work best based on the value the practice will receive vs. the time and other resources it will need to invest to gain access to that information.

Market Strategy

With the market analysis completed, the next step in the marketing plan is to develop a market strategy, which details the broad plan to achieve the practice's objectives with regard to marketing. This may include using the information and data collected to determine which consumers' wants and needs are not being met by the practice or by the competition, or determining areas where new services or different services would capture new markets.[70]

In developing the marketing strategy, the practice needs to identify which segment it is "targeting." The target market is a specific group of consumers who have a want or need for the practice's services or products. For example, a dermatology practice is looking to market its new laser therapy to women and has determined the target age range as 24 to 50 years of age. Target marketing allows the practice to reach, create awareness in, and influence the group of consumers (e.g., in this case, women aged 24 to 50) most likely to select its services while conserving resources and generating greater returns.

Market segmentation – the method of grouping a market into smaller subgroups – is the process of target marketing. Market segments can be geographic (as in a certain region or climate), demographic (by age or race), psychographic (concerning attitudes, behaviors, lifestyles, or loyalty characteristics), or historical (regarding previous customers).

For example, if the practice's services are confined to a specific geographic area, then the target market can be further defined to reflect the number of users of the service within that geographic segment. If an orthopedic practice in Aspen, Colo., is marketing its products and services, it will most likely target its efforts to the surrounding town – the local hospital, employers, ski companies, resorts, hotels, and lodges where injured skiers or family members may return to seek recommendations.

Once target markets are identified, the practice needs to develop a marketing mix that is positioned to be attractive to that segment. The marketing mix enables practices to join together different marketing decision areas, such as products, prices, promotions, and place – also known as the 4Ps – to develop an overall marketing plan.[71]

Products

In medical group practices, products are typically services; with regard to marketing mix and marketing plan development, these services should be used as marketing resources, and a focal point should be differentiation of the practice's services from that of the competition. For example, the orthopedic practice in Aspen may offer a product line that includes orthopedic consultation, radiology services, surgery, and possibly physical therapy or medical massage, in addition to medical equipment such as crutches, bandages, or braces.

Prices

Determining the total cost to the customer is part of the pricing element. Pricing decisions should take into account profit margins and the probable pricing response of competitors. How the practice prices its services is critical because it will have a direct effect on the success of the practice. Pricing strategies and computations can be complex, but the basic rules of pricing are straightforward:

- All prices must cover costs;
- The best and most effective way of lowering prices is to lower costs;
- Prices must reflect the dynamics of cost, demand, changes in the market, and response to competition;
- Prices must be established to ensure sales. Don't price against a competitive operation alone; rather, price to sell;
- Product utility, longevity, maintenance, and end use must be judged continually, and target prices adjusted accordingly; and
- Prices must be set to preserve order in the marketplace.[72]

Many methods of establishing prices are available to practices, among them:

- *Cost-plus pricing* is used mainly by manufacturers. This method ensures that all costs, both fixed and variable, are covered and the desired profit percentage is attained.
- *Demand pricing* is used by practices that sell their services/ products through a variety of sources at differing prices based on demand.
- *Competitive pricing* is used by practices that are entering a market where there is already an established price and it is difficult to differentiate one product from another.
- *Markup pricing* is used mainly by retailers and does not necessarily apply to medical practices. Markup pricing is calculated by adding the desired profit to the cost of the product.[73]

Promotion

Promotion decisions are those related to communicating and selling to potential customers and usually involve selling, sales promotions, advertising, and public relations – with only the latter two applicable to most group practices. A practice's use of promotion is accomplished through communications about the practice to potential customers. Again, think about the orthopedists in Aspen. For promotion they may choose to place their efforts on television or radio advertisements, listings in the phone book, announcements about the practice in the local newspaper, public service announcements, and community service programs.

Place

Place, meaning placement or distribution, refers to decisions regarding market coverage, member selection, logistics, levels of service, and convenience to the customer. Distribution decisions are best made by analyzing competitors to determine the channels they are using and then deciding whether to use the same type of channel or an alternative that may provide the practice with a strategic advantage. The distribution strategy chosen by the practice will also be based on factors in addition to the channels being used by its competition, including pricing strategy and internal resources. For example, perhaps the orthopedic practice's administrator finds that the competition runs advertising in the Saturday newspaper. S/he may choose to run placement of the practice's ad head-to-head on Saturday, or may decide to run the ad on Sunday, or use another completely different media for advertising instead – for example, sponsoring the equipment for a local youth group's ski club or providing the prizes for a downhill race.

Positioning

Although not a part of E. Jerome McCarthy's original 4Ps of the marketing mix, there is a fifth P for practices to consider as well – positioning. A practice's positioning strategy is affected by a number of variables that are closely tied to the motivations and requirements of target customers as well as the actions of primary competitors.

Before a product can be positioned, several strategic questions need to be addressed, such as: How are the practice's competitors positioning themselves (e.g., the region's best at shoulders, arms, and hand surgery)? What specific attributes do the practice's services have that its competitors do not (e.g., radiology in-house)? What customer needs does the practice's service fulfill (e.g., emergency consultation)? Once these questions have been addressed based on market research, the practice executive can then begin to develop a positioning strategy illustrating exactly how it wants its services perceived by both customers and the competition.

Practice Structure and Culture

The marketing plan in general, as well as specific tasks such as the development of the marketing mix, should consider the structure and culture of the practice. Structural features of the practice are formal, usually inflexible, created and maintained by documentation, and contingency centered – they set responsibilities, formal rights, and rewards or punishments on which individual behavior or group action is contingent.[74] The structure determines how the practice is supposed to operate and for what purpose. The culture of the practice, in contrast, is informal, flexible, created and maintained by word of mouth, and ideology centered: it defines good and bad, winning and losing, friends and enemies, and so forth.[75] The cultural characterizations of the practice – people, circumstances, events, objects, facts, processes, and information – are critical for practice decisions and progress. Structure and culture are unique to each practice and shape the image that the practice presents to the community.

The marketing plan for the practice should align with the practice's structure and culture, its style and image, and what makes the practice unique. "Truth in marketing/advertising" is an adage that applies well here. Marketing materials should accurately depict the practice, and the messages utilized should be shared by members of the practice. For example, if the practice has a culture of building relationships with patients, the marketing materials should reflect this, rather than focus on maintaining high efficiency and quick turnaround in seeing patients. The style or image of the practice must be evaluated.

Advertising

The final component of the marketing plan addresses advertising, which relates to the topic of promotion previously discussed. Gone are the days when a practice could "hang out a shingle" and the phone would begin to ring. Health care is an extremely competitive marketplace that requires practices to often rely on innovative advertising practices. Today's practices are, in every sense of the word, "businesses," and they must utilize advertising concepts that were once shunned by the health care industry, such as direct-to-consumer marketing through television and radio advertisements, direct mail, public seminars, creation of Internet Websites or newsletters, and even use of billboards or other signage. The choice of advertising method should be guided by consideration of the following questions:

- What is the source of the practice's current patients?
- What method is optimal for conveying the practice's "message"?
- What method will reach the largest concentration of potential customers?
- What is the cost per unit (i.e., new patient) for this type of method? What is the expected return on investment?
- Is this method ethical in all possible respects?

Once an advertising method has been selected, the practice needs to ensure that the materials designed are written at an appropriate reading level and are clear, concise, and appealing, taking into consideration the population most likely to be served by the practice. Advertising materials, as with all other components of the marketing plan, also need to accurately and honestly portray the practice.

Summary

It is no longer effective to identify target customers and then try to let them know how good the practice is or that the practice wants their business. Instead, the practice must be able to differentiate itself in terms of how it recruits and trains, how it manages people and work, how it uses technology to add value to the customer (in addition to the ways the competition uses it), what new services or products it is offering, how it advertises and promotes these products and services, and more. A marketing plan will assist the practice in accomplishing these goals.

Conclusion

TREMENDOUS AMOUNTS OF DATA are needed to ensure that the Business Operations domain is appropriately managed. Whether it is selecting business partners, developing operational plans, or directing the marketing and communication plans, this domain demands an orientation to and mastery of organizational and analytical skills.

Most financial statements are ultimately broken down to revenues vs. expenses, and many discussions are held over reimbursement rates or the lack thereof. Knowing how to manage this common concern requires an orientation to collecting and analyzing relevant information from multiple sources, discerning the salient data, and making sound decisions based on this information.

The Business Operations domain requires the practice executive to interact with people, but communication cannot be effective without solid organizational and analytical skills. These skills help the executive to manage practice resources and work toward reaching consensus and achieving best performance.

Operating a medical practice is not like managing a hospital, nursing home, or retail store. It requires a special set of technical and professional knowledge and skills that are unheard of by other professions. The diversity and variety of situations that occur in a medical practice make its managers a unique breed. The medical practice executive is expected to have both a general knowledge of many areas as well as a specific capacity to handle detailed information in these areas. An example is the practice executive facilitating a physician-owner board meeting. In that meeting, the group will:

1. Review the monthly and year-to-date financials and budgets (Financial Management);
2. Consider a marketing campaign for launching a new service (Business Operations);
3. Consider another malpractice carrier (Risk Management);
4. Assess the progress made in the electronic medical record project (Information Management);
5. Explore a new patient flow method (Patient Care Systems);
6. Nominate a new board member (Organizational Governance);
7. Hear the Ethics Committee's recommendation on a patient-confidentiality issue (Quality Management); and
8. Evaluate pension plan changes (Human Resource Management).

These topics cover the broad spectrum of medical practice tasks and situations in the *Medical Practice Management Body of Knowledge* performance domains, and require the medical practice executive to understand and apply each of them.

The practice executive requires proficiency and competency in the four general competencies of professionalism, leadership, communication skills, and critical thinking skills. The knowledge and skills needed in the Business Operations domain are critical for the success of both the practice executive and the medical practice. By mastering this domain, the practice executive will be able to apply his or her talents to effectively lead the organization toward success.

Exercises

THESE QUESTIONS have been retired from the ACMPE Essay Exam question bank. Because there are so many ways to handle various situations, there are no "right" answers, and thus, no answer key. Use these questions to help you practice responses in different scenarios.

1. You are an administrator of a large multispecialty medical group practice. During the past 24 months, there has been a drop in work relative value units for physicians and other providers. In two weeks, there is a meeting of the executive committee, and you have been asked to specifically identify the factors that have contributed to the decline and estimate what the impact has been on the medical group.

   What course of action would you take in this situation?

2. You are the administrator of a 10-physician surgical group. A major insurer from which you receive 30 percent of your total revenue has announced that it will reduce reimbursement rates by an average of 25 percent within the next 60 days. You have been instructed by your board of directors to cut your overhead expenses by 10 percent and to ensure that the physicians' distributed compensation does not significantly decrease. The physicians want you to report back to them on how you are going to cut expenses at the next board meeting (in two weeks).

   What course of action would you take in this situation?

3. You are the administrator of a four-physician orthopedic practice in a rural area. The physicians travel to 15 satellite clinics in order to meet the needs of referring physicians and patients. Several physicians believe that they are not seeing a sufficient number of patients to justify their travel time and are considering the elimination of some sites.

   Discuss how you would help the physicians arrive at a decision.

4. You are the administrator of a six-physician, single-specialty medical practice. The practice grew over a period of 20 years, and until two years ago, it was the only practice for this specialty in the immediate and surrounding area. Your service area comprises several small to mid-sized communities. About two years ago, competition to your practice emerged in one of the nearby communities. Additionally, you have become increasingly concerned about the decline in gross revenue resulting from patients transferring out of the practice and the lack of new patient registrations and referrals.

   Describe how you would handle this situation.

5. You are the administrator of a satellite facility for a multispecialty group practice, which is located in a suburb approximately 25 miles from the central facility. The satellite is staffed with eight family practitioners, two nurse practitioners, and rotating specialists from the main facility. The satellite practice serves a different payer mix than the overall medical group. A small multispecialty practice from a neighboring suburb recently opened a new facility within a mile of your site. While your payer contracts are secure, several of the payers have been offering point-of-service products with open provider panels. These products have experienced significant growth. You are concerned that you will lose market share to the competing multispecialty group and have discussed the situation with the physicians at your site.

   Describe how you would further address this situation.

6. You have been the administrator of a successful group practice for five years. However, managed care reimbursement is beginning to erode the income of physicians in your community. Many groups have attempted to reduce their administrative overhead. Several physicians in your group have expressed concern over what they perceive to be high administrative overhead. A physician has told you that several of the physicians feel that the administrative staff should be cut.

   Describe how would you handle this situation.

Notes

1. Reprinted from *MGMA Connexion,* April 2008, with permission of Medical Group Management Association. All rights reserved.
2. Patrick Lencioni, *The Five Dysfunctions of a Team* (San Francisco: Jossey-Bass, 2002).
3. Susan R. Lambreth, *Don't Just Plan – Implement: Steps to Successful Practice Group Plans*, Hildebrandt International Publications. https://www.hildebrandt.com/Documents.aspx?Doc_ID=1938 (accessed Aug. 18, 2005).
4. Ibid.
5. JIAN Tools for Sales, "Components of a Business Plan," www.jian.com/software/business-plan/write-a-business-plan/Components.htm (accessed Aug. 18, 2005).
6. "Elements of a Business Plan," *Entrepreneur.com Magazine,* 2001, www.entrepreneur.com/article/0,4621,287355,00.html (accessed Aug. 18, 2005).
7. Ibid.
8. Ibid.
9. Ibid.
10. JIAN Tools for Sales, "Components of a Business Plan."
11. PlanWare, "White Paper: Writing a Business Plan," www.planware.org/bizplan.htm (accessed Aug. 18, 2005).
12. Austin Ross, Stephen J. Williams, and Ernest J. Pavlock, *Ambulatory Care Management* (Englewood, CO: Medical Group Management Association, 1998), 72.
13. Albert Barnett and Gloria Gilbert Mayer, *Ambulatory Care Management and Practice* (Gaithersburg, MD: Aspen Publishers, 1992), 39–41.
14. Compiled from Medical Group Management Association *Cost Survey for Multispecialty Practices and Cost Survey for Single-Specialty Practices*, 2008 Report Based on 2007 Data.
15. Ibid.

16. Medical Group Management Association *Cost Survey for Multispecialty Practices, 2006 Report Based on 2005 Data* (Englewood, CO: MGMA, 2006), 27.

17. Health Industry Distributors Association, *Strategic Analysis of Physician Office Spending Behavior* (2005), 15.

18. Joseph Mantone, "Trade Wars," *Modern Healthcare* (Sept. 21, 2006), 52.

19. S. Anderson, "In Today's Economy (and Tomorrow's), Strategic Alliances Open Doors to Opportunities," *Orange County Business Journal* 25, no. 4 (Jan. 28-Feb. 3, 2002): 4.

20. John R. Harbison and Peter Pekar, *A Practical Guide to Repeatable Success* (San Francisco: Jossey-Bass, 1998).

21. Timothy Rotarius and Dawn Oetjen, "Dialysis Center Alliances," *Dialysis & Transplantation* 31, no. 3 (2002): 151–154.

22. Ibid.

23. Peter R. Kongstvedt, David W. Plocher, and Jean C. Stanford, "Integrated Health Care Delivery Systems," in *Essentials of Managed Health Care*, 4th ed., ed. Peter R. Kongstvedt (Gaithersburg, MD: Aspen Publishers, 2001), 31–62.

24. Michael K. Rich, "Requirements for Successful Marketing Alliances," *The Journal of Business and Industrial Marketing* 18, no. 4/5 (2003): 447–457.

25. Thomas M. Finn and David A McCamey, "P&G's Guide to Successful Partnerships," *Pharmaceutical Executive* 22, no. 1 (January 2002): 54–60.

26. Rich, "Requirements for Successful Marketing Alliances."

27. Salvatore Parise and Lisa Sasson, "Leveraging Knowledge Management Across Strategic Alliances," *Ivey Business Journal* 66, no. 4 (March/April 2002): 41–47.

28. Kongstvedt, Plocher, and Stanford, "Integrated Health Care Delivery Systems."

29. Peter M. Ginter, Linda E. Swayne, and W. Jack Duncan, *Strategic Management of Health Care Organizations*, 4th ed. (Malden, MA: Blackwell Publishing, 2002), 240.

30. Alan M. Zuckerman, "Strategic Alliances and Joint Ventures: Why Make When You Can Buy?" *Healthcare Financial Management* 59, no. 8 (2005): 122–124.

31. Ibid.

32. Kongstvedt, Plocher, and Stanford, "Integrated Health Care Delivery Systems."

33. Ibid.

34. Ibid.
35. Ibid.
36. Ibid.
37. Ibid.
38. Ibid.
39. Ibid.
40. Ibid.
41. Ibid.
42. Ibid.
43. Ibid.
44. Ibid.
45. Ibid.
46. Rod Aymond and Theodore Hariton, "Regrouping after Disintegration," *Family Practice Management* 7, no. 3 (2000): 37–40.
47. Kriss Barlow and Allison McCarthy, "Due Diligence on the Internal Front Enhances Recruiting Success," *The New England Journal of Medicine* (January/February 2004).
48. Ibid.
49. United States Agency for International Development (USAID), "Due Diligence for Private Enterprise," www.usaid.gov/our_work/global_partnerships (accessed Oct. 17, 2005).
50. Ibid.
51. Ibid.
52. Aymond and Hariton, "Regrouping after Disintegration."
53. Ibid.
54. Ibid.
55. Parise and Sasson, "Leveraging Knowledge Management across Strategic Alliances."
56. Rich, "Requirements for Successful Marketing Alliances."
57. James G. March and Zur Shapira, "Managerial Perspectives on Risk and Risk Taking," *Management Science* 33 (1987): 1404–1418.
58. John Hagedoorn, "Understanding the Rationale of Strategic Technology Partnering: Interorganizational Modes of Cooperation and Sectoral Differences," *Strategic Management Journal* 14 (1993): 371–385; B. Kogut, "Joint Ventures: Theoretical and Empirical Perspectives," *Strategic Management Journal* 9 (1988): 319–332.

59. Oliver E. Williamson, "Credible Commitments: Using Hostages to Support Exchange," *American Economic Review* 73 (1983): 519–540; Oliver E. Williamson, *The Economic Institutions of Capitalism* (New York: Free Press, 1985).

60. Anderson, "In Today's Economy (and Tomorrow's), Strategic Alliances Open Doors to Opportunities."

61. Ibid.

62. Clarkson Centre for Ethics & Board Effectiveness, "Redefining the Corporation: Publications: Principles of Stakeholder Management," www. Mgmt.utoronto.ca/~stake.Publications.htm.

63. Ibid.

64. Ibid.

65. Ibid.

66. Ibid.

67. Louis E. Boone and David L. Kurtz, *Contemporary Marketing Wired*, 3rd ed. (New York: Dryden Press, 1998).

68. Michael E. Porter, *Competitive Strategy* (New York: Free Press, 1980).

69. American Marketing Association, "Marketing Definitions," www.marketingpower.com/ (1995; accessed Sept. 9, 2005).

70. Meir Liraz, "Managing a Small Business," www.liraz.com/marketing.htm (1998; accessed Sept. 10, 2005).

71. Ibid.

72. "Market Strategies," *Entrepreneur.com Magazine*, www.entrepreneur.com/article/0,4621,270370,00.html (2004; accessed Aug. 18, 2005).

73. Ibid.

74. Gather the People, "Training Guide #7: Organizational Structure and Culture," www.gatherthepeople.org/Downloads/007_STRUCTURE_CULTURE.pdf (2004; accessed Sept.13, 2005).

75. Ibid.

Index

Note: (ex.) indicates exhibit.